Running

SUCKS!

Lose Pounds & Inches Using the
Effortless Exercise Method,
5-Second Flat Belly Secret &
5-Minute Miracle Exercises

By Jennifer Jolan

and

Rich Bryda

LESS WEIGHT AWAITS YOU!

COPYRIGHT AND TRADEMARK NOTICES

TABLE OF CONTENTS

1 How To Lose Weight Spinning In A Circle   1
   Like Kids

2 Introduction to the Running Sucks Method: 17
   The Effortless Exercise Method for Women -
   How to Lose Weight Faster & Easier Without
   Needing to Go to a Gym

3 The Four Concepts Of "Effortless Exercise"   23

4 Mini-Workouts   41

5 The 4-Minute Workout   45

6 The Exercises   51

7 A Premier 5-Minute Miracle Exercise That   55
   Says "No" To The Stairstepper And "Yes" To
   Fat Loss

8 Bumping Up Your Game   65

9 Three Exercises For That Curvy, Feminine   71
   Hourglass Figure

10 How To Do Hitt "Running" For Successful   77
   Weight Loss

11 Doing Other Exercises Not Mentioned Here   83

12 The Running Sucks Effortless Exercise System   85
   Summary

13 Other Stomach-Enhancers   87

14 The 1-Minute T-Tap   99

15 Concluding Thoughts For Running Sucks   101

   References   105

1

HOW TO LOSE WEIGHT SPINNING
IN A CIRCLE LIKE KIDS

Before we get into the main ideas and exercises of Running Sucks I wanted to share with you a simple, but crazy sounding, bonus exercise that really sounds ludicrous and unbelievable.

We accept that this sounds far-fetched. Just hear us out. After that, what harm will it do to actually test it out? So here it goes...

We're going to explain how you can spin around in circles (just as kids love to do) in order to help you change yourself in three unexpected ways:

1. You'll lose weight!

2. You'll re-energize your body!

3. Your overall health should improve!

Yes, I know it seems kind of weird and strange. Please keep an open mind. Sometimes some of the most obvious things are overlooked.

For example, I recently saw taco shells for sale where the bottom "folded" edges were *flat* so the taco wouldn't fall over on the plate and spill out. Why didn't anyone think of this obvious answer decades ago? No, taco shells aren't the healthiest food around it's an example of things that are right in front of us that nobody considered... until somebody considered it. Then it seems easy and obvious.

Spinning, just as kids do it, is one of those things that seem obvious once you understand what really takes place when you do it. Surprising, but true. I'm amazed it hasn't been part of a healthy workout regimen for ages. Hopefully it will be now.

I'll explain the logic and rationale behind spinning. I'll show you why spinning around actually works for the health benefits that I just mentioned. And, if you still don't believe me after all that you've read, then, I simply challenge you to spin around (as I outline) for 10 to 14 days and prove or disprove it to yourself.

That's not much to ask, is it?

How I Learned About This

This isn't something I invented. I like to read. I read just about anything and everything when it comes to health, exercise, nutrition, or other strange things that make me curious. My readers and my own family benefit from any tool I can add to my healthy arsenal so I stay on top of things closely.

How I learned about spinning was purely accidental. The source that triggered it all came, of all places, from my reading about Sufi Muslims living in Turkey. They are called "*Whirling Dervishes.*"[1]

The spinning around thing that they did fascinated me. I *had* to know more about "why" they did it. The more I read about them and their spinning practice, I began to understand not just why *they* did it, but also why the actual spinning itself produced the effect they sought.[2]

I won't get into the religious aspect of it all. That's unnecessary for our purposes here. I will, however, say that the Sufi Muslims spin around until they reach an ecstatic state of mind as a show of love and a drama of their faith.

That is the "why-they-do-it" part of this. That doesn't account for any health benefits, however.

This is what caught my eye the most the more I learned, read, and saw of them in my research of the Whirling Dervishes: *All of them* were thin, showed amazing energy and stamina, and were youthful looking (compared to their actual ages).

I'll Take It for a Spin Myself!

So I thought to myself "Hmm, okay, what the heck. I'll spin around and see what the big deal is about." I did it. Just once.

Wow... was *that* quite an experience.

I'm glad I was alone! I nearly knocked over a lamp after spinning around 20 times. I had to sit and then lie down on my couch to normalize myself. I rested and felt normal after a few minutes. Most important for our purposes though is that I also felt energized.

More than usual. And I'm a person with lots of energy due to the lifestyle I lead.

Again, this really was something new. As I said, I exercise often and I feel energized from exercising, but *this was a different type of energy* that I felt. I had a tingling sensation feeling in my head and heart. A lightness that's hard to explain was there too.

I felt more alive than before. I felt good!

I wanted more. This was too good to stop now. I needed to take it to the extreme to see what the fuss was about. I always want to push things to the limit to find out as much as possible.

So, I spun around again... this time 15 times. I didn't want to get too dizzy. I spun around and on my final spin I just spun right onto my couch lying down right away. I was kind of delirious with excitement.

Like a child with a new toy. Or like the feeling after a fun ride at an amusement park.

It's a good thing nobody could see what I was doing. Let's face it; it's weird to see a grown woman spinning around like a little kid.

In mulling over everything, spinning around those 15 times did feel like too much for me. Still, I wasn't going to let that stop me. I spun some more. By the time I stopped doing the spins, 30 minutes had passed. I must have done 10 to 15 sets of spins and I never did fewer than 10 spins each time.

More Research Was in Order

That's how I began this quest to see why the spinning did what it did. I also wanted to know more about the health effects. Did spinning help me or do something I'd rather not have done?

If the spinning did contribute to the Sufi's thin waistlines then exactly how did that occur? I'm positive spinning didn't burn more calories than other traditional exercises. In fact, I suspected that spinning burned very few calories, period.

I wanted to know what was going on inside when I spun around. I wanted to know what gave me the uplifting sensations as well as how those spins affected my weight and well-being.

Findings from Research

Honestly, after that first day, I was hooked. I devoted

myself to doing the spins each day. And I wanted to know more about what I was getting myself into. So I dove into doing more research.

I ended up learning some fascinating things.

For example, I learned that those Whirling Dervishes would spin hundreds of times non-stop. By over-spinning, they'd create a huge burst of ecstatic energy that put them into an almost delirious state of mind.

Note: I never do more than 20 spins in a set and you shouldn't either. Stop after 20 and rest for at least one minute... *Always!*

I wasn't after the ecstatic different state of mind thing. I like to keep my senses as I'm sure you do too. I wanted the health benefits, especially since I sometimes get a little sluggish in the mid-afternoon.

But there was something else that I found out. Even though the Whirling Dervishes got huge bursts of energy, they would also have their energy come crashing down within a few hours. I experienced this too. This is *not good* in my opinion. I didn't want a boost only to come down lower than I began... like what sugar does to us.

I wanted a nice even, all-day energy-boost. I didn't want to have an energy-boost that was followed by a state of tiredness or exhaustion. Fortunately for me, I never went above 20 spins at a time because who knew? Maybe I'd throw up or something. I just didn't know. This was all new to me and I was testing various things. So I put my heart into spinning, but I still kept limits.

More Findings

I felt great, had an extra bounce to my step and had the energy of a 4-year old child without having an energy crash by doing too many spins as the whirling dervishes do.

Happily I also noticed I had become more toned than

usual.

Keep in mind I've always been in good shape because that is my job. I've always thought "outside the box." I've always done things my own way when it comes to training and dieting for weight loss and health. If the whole world does something (such as extended aerobics, ugh!), then probably there's a better, easier, and healthier way to approach it.

Understand that I already had a grab-bag of "tricks" and "tweaks" to exercising and dieting that gave people miracle results.

But the spins – what began for me as a way to boost my energy levels – soon proved to be another weight loss "trick" I could add to my arsenal. But I wanted to be sure. I thought I better find out if this really works for weight loss for most people and not just for me.

This was when I approached some of my weight loss clients and friends and explained the spins to them. Besides the laughing, along with the "you're crazy" looks when I mentioned all this to them, I made them do it.

It was my feeling that, "Geez, if kids do this naturally, what harm could spinning do to grown women?" The proof is in the pudding as they say. Are you interested in my clients' results? There was 100% success with only a few bumps along the road.

The Successes

After 14 days of spinning, all the women experienced one or more of these results: had more energy, felt better, lost a few pounds (some more than others), acted more youthful, and even looked better.

> **Note:** Think about all that. Even if my clients didn't lose weight, spinning would still be awesome for all the other benefits they experienced. I consider any

weight loss an *extra* benefit of spinning.

Are you going to lose 10+ pounds in two weeks from spinning alone? No. That won't happen.

My first group of readers loved the spinning and they got great results. That was all I needed to hear and I released this information to all of my other readers. I've gotten hundreds of positive emails from people who have read this and tried out the spins.

The Few Bumps in the Road Are Simple to Cross

There were a few bumps along the way and it's my duty to share those with you too. The feedback I've received from some of the women shows that perhaps you should ease into doing the spins. In other words, don't attempt to do 20 spins your first time. Build-up to 20 and use 20 spins as your goal.

> Note: You'll build up quickly. You should be able to do 20 spins easily in less than two weeks.

Why should you build up to twenty spins? Based off the feedback, some of the women became too dizzy and had a hard time getting normalized from the dizziness. They simply overdid the spinning. It was too much, too soon and they were unaccustomed. Their body/mind link couldn't keep up with too many spins.

A few women even emailed me that they got sick from nausea. (There are solutions! I'll tell you about those in a few moments.)

The women who got too dizzy and the few women who got sick did end up getting used to spinning within one to two weeks. They didn't give up and I was proud. They were rewarded for their persistence with better health and weight loss. They love spinning now! There was a happy ending even for those few problem cases.

Some Background on Your Body's Reaction to Spinning

Before I get to the outline of how you should spin, I want to explain some of what I found out about the dynamics of why spinning helps people lose weight and gain energy. Also, there is a simple explanation as to why spinning actually makes you younger at a "cellular level."

It all centers around your *endocrine system*.[3]

Your endocrine system consists of seven glands:

- The pineal gland

- The pituitary gland

- The thyroid gland

- The thymus

- The adrenal glands

- The pancreas

- The reproductive glands (testes in men, ovaries in women)

Your endocrine system is vital because it controls your metabolism. Metabolism is the key to either weight gain or weight loss. Your metabolism regulates your growth and development, alters your hormone levels (*extremely vital*), and plays a part in your mood.

Staying Level

Your endocrine system controls your overall well-being in that it helps keep your body in a constant state of *homeostasis*,[4] or in layman's terms, your endocrine system wants you to stay on an "even keel." You want this for the most part. You never want to be too hungry, too cold, too hot, too lazy, too energetic, and so on.

With rare exceptions you want to feel as though you're in control and you're doing just fine in every way.

Many times in life we want to feel more extreme, and many times in life we accept those feelings as natural. It's natural and healthy to feel sadness at the loss of a friend or family member. It's natural and healthy to feel elation when something good happens to you such as paying off a big debt or seeing a child's accomplishment.

But none of us want those extreme feelings to last forever or we couldn't function in our other duties.

If sadness takes over long after a sad event ends, we find it difficult to get the energy to work or to be secure and joyful with family whom we love. If we are too energetic at all times we have difficulty sleeping well because our thoughts are "racing."

Our endocrine system is monitoring us constantly and is the reason we go from normal to extremes and also why we can return from the extremes to normal. (We return from the extremes when our endocrine system is functioning well.) Our endocrine system secretes whatever hormone our body needs at the time in an attempt to maintain a normal, healthy level of living. It's almost like a beautiful ballet act that constantly goes on inside our bodies without us really being aware of it most of the time.

I realize you don't want to be bored with anatomy details, but I wanted to mention the background behind it all.

Those seven glands I mentioned earlier are energy centers for your body. The cell signals revolve in place at each of the seven locations. They do this *in a circular* motion. When I say *circular* you probably are beginning to realize why *spins* can affect our endocrine system.

When cell signals sent by our endocrine system are revolving in place, the signals either revolve fast, slow, or somewhere in-between. This is important because when they are revolving fast, you're in good health and have lots of energy. Everything is going good with your body.

When they are revolving too slowly, you aren't in good health and you don't have much energy. Too slowly means that you generally just don't feel good.

Again, our goal is to be somewhere near the middle most of the time, but that doesn't seem to be the case if you look at others walking down the street and if you listen to others talk about the way they feel. Basically, most people aren't at optimal health. They're closer to poor health. Obviously this manifests itself in lack of energy and obesity.

Their endocrine systems are overworked and overwhelmed

Spinning the News for Good

The good news is, spinning speeds up your endocrine systems ability to send cell signals.

Repeated spinning daily helps to reset your revolving speed upwards. This is good for your health, good for your energy, and good for weight loss!

I hope I explained all of that clearly enough without throwing too many boring details. I want you to understand that spinning can have a powerful effect to alter your health, energy, and weight positively. Now that you know the reasoning behind spinning benefits, let's move on.

Oops, I Left Out Important Information...

I got so caught up in my excitement about spinning that I left out an important piece of information. This comes up more than I expected as I explain to readers about the benefits of spinning.

Note that you can spin either way: clockwise or counter-clockwise. The Whirling Dervishes spin counter-clockwise. Me? Personally, I prefer to spin in a clockwise direction. It just feels more comfortable. But either way, it doesn't matter which way you spin. Try both ways and see which direction you're most comfortable with.

If you want to see how the Whirling Dervishes spin around, just do a Google search on them and go to the many images and videos you'll find.

When you watch the videos you'll see that they tilt their heads while they spin. *I do not want you to do that.* Remember, they're doing this to get extremely dizzy to the point of delirium. This not only can make you sick to your stomach and make your head spin, but it's simply too much and overflows your equilibrium *and* your endocrine system's mechanics.

You're not doing this to achieve delirium – you're spinning for better health and weight loss.

Keep your head straight up like normal. Don't tilt your head... keep it straight. Another thing you may see the Whirling Dervishes do that I don't recommend is they hold their arms against their chest when they start spinning. Don't do this either.

For your arms, put them out as if they were airplane wings: straight out at shoulder level. Then just start spinning around like kids do it. It's fun!

Your Spinning Routine

Above, I described the correct way to spin around. Head straight up and your arms out like airplane wings. Now, here's how you should start out spinning.

Day 1

Begin your first day with spinning around just five times.

11

Faster is not necessarily better, but your goal should be to spin around on the faster side as long as you remain fairly comfortable with the speed. Five times is a base level to try. If you really want to see the "real" effects of spinning, try 15 to 20 spins.

If you're hesitant and don't want to risk extreme dizziness or nausea, just spin five times on your first set of spins. I don't want you to have a rough first time and be afraid to spin in the future.

Once you do this, think through how you feel. Any problems with completing your goal? How did it go? What is your body telling you?

You goal is this and only this: spin only until you are *slightly dizzy*. That is your only goal for each set of spins. That is all you need to do to benefit from spinning and improve your health, increase your energy, and probably lose some weight. The slight dizziness means you affected your equilibrium some, but you didn't overdo things the first time.

> **Note:** Excess dizziness can make you feel *not-so-good* the rest of the day. Obviously.

Just do yourself a favor and trust me. Take it easy and ease into it. Start with five spins and rest *at least* a minute before trying to do more, such as a second set of spins.

Pace yourself and take a real inventory the first time. If five spins didn't really affect you and you're not close to being slightly dizzy, try ten or more spins in a row on your next set.

Keep repeating this until you've done at least fifty total spins.

Remember, this is just day one. I want your body and you to get a "feel" for spinning. If you need a few minutes between each set of spins, take a few minutes. If five spins didn't do anything for you, do more. How many? Use your good judgment and guess. Pace yourself while taking constant inventory of your body and mind. Practice.

Remember:

- Slightly dizzy

- Slightly dizzy

- Slightly dizzy

That's what you want.

Watch TV, Lose Weight

When you watch TV, there are usually 15-20 minutes of commercials during each hour of programming. A good idea is to do your spinning during commercials, if you watch a lot of TV. You could easily get in one or two spin cycles during each commercial break and a minimum of eight sets during an hour of TV.

It's simple to fit these in; you have no excuses!

After your first set, use your own good judgment on how long to rest and how many spins you should do for the next set. If you got really dizzy with just five spins, then consider taking a long rest and doing three spins the next time. But whatever you do, don't quit.

For almost every person who follows this outline, their body usually adjusts to the spins within two to seven days... and 14 days at the latest. It rarely takes people two weeks.

That can happen though if they had problems with some extreme dizziness to begin with.

If you're one who likes to jump into the deep end of the pool right away, you're more than welcome to just go ahead and spin around 15 to 20 times on your first try. But I must warn you... you may get really dizzy to the point of being nauseous and throwing up.

My fear with you doing that is you may quit the program right away without giving it an honest chance if that happens to you.

So again, you've been warned!

Seriously, please use common sense. Listen to your body and mind. Pay attention to how your body reacts and adjust accordingly with either less or more spins per set, whether slower or faster spins, and more or less rest between each set of spins. Just remember the most important goal with spins: spin to the point where you get *slightly dizzy*... or at most, do 20 spins during a set.

By paying attention to your reaction to each set of spins, you'll generally know where that point is. Just know this: You're not in a race. This is something you can and should do for the rest of your life, every day. It's that important.

Even if it takes you two weeks to get used to spinning, so be it. Your body, your health, and your lower healthcare bills will thank you for it over the years.

Days Two through Five

Gradually challenge your body more as time goes by. Complete more spins per set, spin faster, and rest less between each set. Build up to what your body reacts to well.

Note: Each person is different so, as with most routines, don't get caught up with the numbers. The only number that is important is the total number of spins you do each day. Eventually you'll want to build up to 100+ spins a day.

But that may take a week or two or more for some people. And *that's fine*. Progress is more important than speedy progress. Now, understand that 100+ total spins each day is your ultimate goal.

However you go about this is fine, I just don't want you to quit during the first two weeks. I am positive that if you do the spins for two weeks, you will be so happy with the results and you'll be more than happy to do these spins daily for a long, long time.

How I Spin Each Day

My daily spin routine is simple. I usually spin 20 times for each set. I do 10 (more if I can) sets daily for a total of 200 or more spins each and every day. That probably is on the excessive side, but I enjoy doing them. They make me feel awesome and help tone me up. (My children love to spin with me also!)

I usually do three sets of 20 spins right when I wake up. After that, I just do them whenever I get the chance throughout the day. Basically I do them when I have room to spin, and about 30 seconds of free time. I don't feel guilty watching TV here and there throughout the day because I get in a lot of spins during TV commercials also.

So, I personally aim for 10 sets a day. I've turned them into a habit, so I don't need to think about it. I just do them when I get a chance. This makes it easy since I don't have to stress out about how many sets I've done and how many more I need to do.

I simply have the habit of doing my first three sets when I wake up and then the rest will come throughout the day whenever possible.

Final Thoughts

I think of this when I think of the life-changing power spinning around in circles has for people: I don't gamble, but imagine knowing of a casino where the blackjack dealer showed his hand before you made your move and didn't care how many times you beat him.

When would you stop going there? I hope your answer to that question would be a resounding, *"Never!"* (Assuming you're sane, that is!)

Well, that is a *perfect* analogy on the power of spinning around like a child.

Once you discover the powerful health, energy, and weight loss benefits of spinning around in a circle like a child by practicing it daily, why on Earth would you ever stop doing them?

But guess what? I've had clients who lost quite a bit of weight and had a huge increase in energy and lots of other health benefits, and yet, they quit doing them. I cannot fathom why. Please, don't you be one of them. With that said, it's time for you to do some spins.

And, up next, it's time for you to learn about the concepts and exercises that entail Running Sucks!

2

INTRODUCTION TO THE RUNNING SUCKS METHOD: THE EFFORTLESS EXERCISE METHOD FOR WOMEN - HOW TO LOSE WEIGHT FASTER & EASIER WITHOUT NEEDING TO GO TO A GYM

Thank you for getting our *Running Sucks* book. A mere month from now, you'll have seen and proven to yourself that getting this was a smart investment. You will not have agonized trying to jog off the pounds (which is extremely inefficient actually.)

More important, your mirror won't lie!

A month from now you'll have a totally new body. Yes, new thighs, new hips, and a new flatter belly! The way you achieve this is certainly not by jogging, but by using a few revolutionary concepts that will be brand new to many readers.

These concepts incorporate the core of a "new you."

In getting that new body, you won't sweat much, and perhaps not at all. We prefer not to sweat, right? Plus, you really don't even need to go to the gym. But still, you'll be getting a more toned and leaner body. Then, each month after that, as you continue using this system your body will keep improving and looking better.

> **Note:** Before I go further, if strict weight loss is your overriding goal, I want to make clear that the fastest way to lose weight is through dieting. For that, I highly recommend you check out our 10-Hour Coffee Diet and 1-Day Diet books.

Different is Good

I have no doubt that you will find this is a bit different from other material on the subject of exercise. I'm writing this specifically for busy women who hate running... but those who still feel they need to run (a little) in order to lose weight. This book isn't written for serious runners who run for enjoyment.

I consider running a necessary evil. Before you're done here I believe you will agree with me.

You will soon find that running isn't complicated. Running doesn't need hundreds of pages of pointless information just to fill up pages for the average person. Even though an exercise or two that follow have the word *running* in their name, they don't feel like running and that are about as far from the traditional "running" as one can possibly get.

In a Nutshell

What you do need to know are a few important things. I want you to maximize every second you put into exercising. I want you to gain the most benefit possible in the least amount of time and effort.

If you take these tips seriously and implement them faithfully, you'll be greatly rewarded. I promise.

What I present for you is simple and clear. Be warned, however, it may not necessarily be easy for *you*. But all I ask is that you just understand that running is exercise and running does require some effort. "Nothing ventured, nothing gained," "no pain no gain," and all that. Except here, your pain is reduced tremendously! To be clear, this book contains isn't all about running or jogging.

In fact, it is more about exercises, and an exercise methodology, that are far more efficient for fat loss than jogging.

I set out to design *Running Sucks* so you stop dreading running. In addition, I want you to be able to get your running over with as fast as possible. Let's face it... your body may be enhanced by running, but running isn't your life. Running for you is a means to an end (better fitness, reduced weight) but you don't live to run.

Let me prepare you for what's ahead. It may shock you, but in a good way. It is possible that you may be able to run *in your home* and definitely *without* a treadmill! Yeah, I thought it sounded impossible and weird too when I first discovered the secrets behind *Running Sucks*, but you'll see I am correct.

Why do people fail to maintain their exercise routine?

1. Exercise is often inconvenient

2. Exercise is often a hassle to fit into our busy lives.

To help you achieve your fitness goals and still reduce the problems associated with running as much as possible, I set out to design *Running Sucks* to not only be effective for you, but also so you can fit exercise easily into your busy schedule. I achieve success from my writing when my readers succeed.

It is in *my* best interest to maximize *your* success.

Some Goals

I designed *Running Sucks* with three primary goals:

1. Your routines have to be quick (5 minutes or less in most cases)

2. Everything needs to be doable on the cheap (no need for a gym membership or buying a treadmill)

3. Everything here must be convenient for any reader (all can be done at home or close by).

So, keep all that in mind. Together we will focus on just the *top* key factors of exercise (and running) that will get you the most results in the least amount of time.

Stop dreading the track or treadmill. Reduce your running (and exercise) time and in many instances, effort... and increase the time you can spend doing other things. That's what life is all about.

The Best Part of this Effortless Exercise Method

The great part of this exercise system is the convenience. You can do most or all of the exercises at home during TV commercials. This means that you'll save money by not needing a gym membership. You'll save time by not having to go to and from a gym.

And because of the convenience of being able to work out from home, you'll also be more likely to stick with the program. In taking care of and improving our bodies, consistency ensures success.

And months and years of consistency helps ensure long-term health... and a great looking body.

Speaking of TV, as you'll soon see, I actually encourage you to use this method of working out during TV commercials. So to go against the grain of most trainers and body-strengthening authors, I say "Heck, go watch TV!" I'm not going to fight you on that. All I want is your time during the commercials.

That's not asking much, is it?

Correcting Common Wrongs

Throughout this book, there are some simple concepts that I want to ingrain in you. A lot of what most people know about getting firmer and sexier is completely wrong.

Too many programs and concepts out there do nothing more than this: they make the simple complicated. I don't know if that's to intentionally confuse people in order to sell books and magazines or whether it is unintentional.

As for me, *I promise you*, if you just go this route with me and give this system and exercises a try for one month you'll never go back to the typical weight resistance or and cardio workouts.

Those do nothing more than waste your time and resources.

Plus, they give you such little marginal gain – and often they *reduce* your possible gains – that from this point forward your entire outlook on improving your body will dramatically change for the better.

Additionally, you won't have had to jog ever again!

You'll learn things that fulfill your wants and needs such as:

- If you want smaller and firmer hips… I'll show you how to do that in a month.

- If you want an hourglass figure... done, just give my system a month.

- Nicer thighs and hips and a toned belly?… done in a month (obviously this depends on your starting point).

I've built flexibility into the system to allow you to choose what you want. If you want to skip directly working your legs, okay then do so. Not a problem. It's your body. I'm not trying to force my ideal body onto you and your goals.

You'll find cardio exercises, leg exercises, arm exercises, waist and hips exercises, home exercises, gym exercises, outdoor exercises, easy exercises, harder exercises, and exercises for cellulite.

Pick and choose what you need most.

Note: The first part of this book's program is effortless exercise, but there's more after that! I want to over-give with answers that will last you a lifetime. So, in addition to offering you a literal "Effortless Exercise System," you'll later find several additional exercises and methods that boost your body's low-fat, high-energy state and make you look better than you've looked in years!

3
THE FOUR CONCEPTS OF "EFFORTLESS EXERCISE"

The Effortless Exercising System is built on a foundation of four pillars. The good news is that by learning and practicing those four core pillar concepts, you can't help but to get a nicer looking body.

In fact, you should write out and tape the four concepts onto your wall as a friendly reminder.

Straight to the Point!

Now, before I begin, I just want to say that I absolutely hate reading books that are full of page after page of fluff information that tells me nothing. All fluff but no stuff!

I just want to yell at the author, "Get to the point!"

I keep that in mind while writing. I'm going to get right to the point in this book. I have no doubt that you value your time as much as I value mine. I'm not going to waste your time by forcing you to read pages and pages of useless information just to get to the "good stuff."

I don't see the value in long books that are long just to fill pages.

As you saw from the price, I don't see the value of

expensive books either. Still, personally I'd rather pay more for something that is short and amazingly informative than something that is long, boring, and full of fluff and impractical information.

The value is in the quality of information. Here, that information is being presented clearly in as quick a manner as possible. This program is designed for women to get a more toned, sexier looking body.

You can do these exercises 20 to 30 minutes a day (5 or less minutes at a time), six days a week, during TV commercials. You can also perform mini-workouts throughout the day for one month to transform your body and get awesome results. All without jogging and all without any of the traditional, boring, long gym sessions you see others doing for fewer results.

If you want to put in more time than that, by all means, go for it. As with anything, the more work you put in daily (within reason), the better your results.

But as long as you follow the four core concepts, you can put in an almost limitless amount of time into exercising each day

Do you need to follow all four of the core concepts? No. But, by following all four core concepts, you'll get better results, faster.

Okay, let's get started.

Main Concept #1: Imprinting is the Key

Neural Imprinting[5] is the basic concept to use when exercising in order to get results with what seems to be little effort (effortless).

Neural Imprinting, or the specific and formal aspect we'll discuss here called the *Neural Impulse Development Method* (NIDM),[6] revolves around the ability to efficiently develop your neural pathway between your brain, your muscles, and your cells.

By building up and strengthening the connection pathway between these three things, your body will magically get more toned, firm up, and lose excess weight with less effort.

For many women, because of the efficiency and strengthening of the pathway, it's much easier to develop a more feminine toned look without gaining bigger "guy" muscles in the process. I am just going to assume you don't want big "guy muscles."

Neuroscientists call this neural efficiency the *Hebb Rule*.[7]

The rule says the following:

The persistence or repetition of a reverberatory activity tends to induce lasting cellular changes that add to its stability. When an axon of cell A is near enough to excited a cell B and repeatedly or persistently takes part in firing it, some growth process or metabolic change takes place in one or both cells such that A's efficiency, as one of the cells firing B, is increased.

Basically what it is saying is that "Cells that fire together, wire together. Simultaneous activation of cells leads to pronounced increases in synaptic strength between the cells."

In other words, if you do something (whatever it may be, say a pushup or pull-up or even non-exercise movements), the next time you do that same movement it will be easier due to the Hebb Rule and increased neural efficiency.

Your body becomes more and more sculpted as you build up the neural efficiency.[8]

This is why the main concept #3 (that we discuss later) is all about doing a lot of "fresh" repetitions (this doesn't mean a lot of repetitions per set) and main concept #4 is about high frequency of movements; are two of the foundation concepts you must take to heart in order to get toned and slimmer... easier and in less time.

Now, that's not to say that you can't get a better-looking body by not following these core concepts.

You can, but you just won't do it in an efficient and fast manner. On top of that, you'll probably be in a constant plateau and never truly improve your body if you avoid using at least a couple of the four core concepts mentioned here.

In conclusion, the Neural Impulse Development Method is just one key to making this all work. Combined with the other key concepts below; guess what? You'll look incredible.

Later I'll outline some sample workouts as examples of what you can do to put this all together into something easy and doable for you. The best concepts and ideas won't do you any good if you can't easily do them.

Simplicity breeds activity, which breeds consistency, which breeds success.

Before going to the next main concept, I want you to think of your nervous system as a coach. Your system is coaching your muscles, your cells, and your nerve impulses to work together in an efficient, coordinated manner to get the most out of the team effort.

How can you expect to get more toned and lose fat when your muscles, your cells, and your nerves don't work together in coordination if they're all doing their own thing?

Using reason, it becomes clear that the more coordinated and the more efficient your body and its components work together, the more you'll progress.

Main Concept #2: Avoid F&F

Most people think that totally trashing their muscle fibers to exhaustion and going all out each set is the best way to stimulate weight loss and toning.

That is simply *wrong*! Generally speaking, you need to avoid both Fatigue and muscular Failure (F&F).

A complete beginner is someone in who *any* type of exercise method used would cause her to initially tone up a little and lose some weight. But if you train to failure (failure to do another rep or complete exhaustion during cardio) you will find that it is the biggest obstacle holding back progress to the majority of you and everybody else exercising.

Fortunately, many women don't feel the need to exercise to failure.

We find that most men who begin lifting weights do this. Still, I don't ever want you to work out to the point of not being able to do another repetition on a set of exercise because not only will you feel bad and achy; but doing that "fries" your central nervous system.

When you burn out your central nervous system, you decrease its neurological efficiency.

One good way to see this is to think of a sports team. What if you trained a team to act individually? Instead of giving a strong team effort with all the players doing their job, each player does his own thing without any thought to what's best for the team.

A team like that wouldn't win anything regardless of how great its players are.

That's an example of an inefficient team. And training to failure – or close to it – does the same thing to your central nervous system (CNS).[9] It causes your CNS to become inefficient by burning it out.

Your central nervous system basically kind of shuts down a bit and says "No, I'm not going to give you all I got. I can't handle it anymore. I need a break. But since you're too dumb to realize that I'm being overworked, I'm going to make you feel tired and achy in order for you to get the message."

Intensity is good and vitally important, but intensity has to be controlled and managed.

Reckless intensity, such as doing all sets to failure all the time, is out of control intensity that has a huge ripple effect on all your other aspects of training. The key to training is to master the set because doing sets wrong will have a domino effect that dictates how and when you train.

So, always keep in mind, training to failure and complete fatigue causes your progress to grind to a halt. It's just too much.

The body needs to be stimulated – not destroyed.

A Rep Example

If for example you can do an exercise for 10 reps, do anywhere from 3 to 6 reps for each set instead of the full 10 reps you could have done. I'll get into the dynamic of how this change leads to improved toning soon.

The key for this chapter is to remember to manage and avoid fatigue and muscular failure. Don't seek it out as something good. Getting completely tired after every set for hours each week will make your progress stall out because of the extra time you'll need to rest between workouts in order to refresh your body and muscles again so that they can perform appropriately.

This results in less stimulation, overall, for your body.

Someone who manages to avoid fatigue with each set will be able to work out more often and do more sets and more total reps. Extra stimulation provides for more toning and weight loss gains. Failure and fatigue end up making you fall behind over the long run.

You won't be able to firm up or lose weight, except in the very beginning. You don't want to be that person stuck in a plateau for years. No doubt you've seen people who exercise a lot but never progress (maybe you are that person – I hope not!).

The more you work out to the point of complete exhaustion and fatigue, the longer it will take you to reach your goals.

You'll just end up falling behind and not being able to lose weight or tone up as fast as possible. So, pay attention to your fatigue at the end of each set (including cardio sets) and make sure to avoid all-out fatigue as much as possible.

Note: Later I'll show you how to control fatigue smartly with Tabata and HIIT.

You do this by avoiding muscular failure.

Main Concept #3: L.R. +L.S. + S.R.T. = N.E.

The formula is:

Low Reps + Lots of Sets + Short Rest Times = Neurological Efficiency

The result, *Neurological Efficiency*, equates to more juice to your body as you work out and your workouts become far more efficient. More efficiency equates to you being firmer and more toned.

Here's the deal.

Doing high reps (long distance jogging for example) is either neurologically inefficient or it burns out your Nervous System, fast. Many times both occur.

Even if you're doing an exercise that is a light weight for you, cut it off before doing a lot of reps (repetitions). For example, if you can lift a 20-pound dumbbell for 10 reps (10 reps being failure and you can't do any additional reps even if you wanted to), if you followed what I have to say, you'd *never* (or rarely) do more than 5 to 6 reps per set.

Instead of getting the stimulation of your muscles from going to failure which burns out your Nervous System and weakens your neurological efficiency, you'd stimulate your Nervous System with more sets and shorter rest times from these "easy" 5 to 6 rep sets of 20 pounds.

That's just an example using weights. You don't need to use weights if you don't want to. Use the same principle for exercises that don't involve weights, too.

Inconsistency Leads to Failure

A big reason why people don't get results from working out is because they're inconsistent. A big reason for inconsistency is the hassle of going to and from the gym.

It's much easier just to work out at home.

Back to low reps. The key thing in doing low reps not to muscular failure is you keep your Nervous System fresh and able to recover from all the stimulation. You'll let the overall volume (lots of sets) and short rest times take care of your ability to tone and lose fat.

Later on, I mention how you can do one set every so often throughout the day. In this regard, you won't have short rest times. In fact, you'll have really long rest times of maybe an hour or more before doing another set.

This appears to be a contradiction, but it isn't.

What I mean by "short rest times" is if you're doing a workout that has multiple sets, you need short rest times between sets. So, when I talk about short rest times, I mean within a work out.

Later in this book you'll get plenty of examples to use yourself or to work off of to develop your own workouts. It's best that you develop your own workouts instead of following a cookie-cutter program because 1-size-fits-all programs won't work for everyone. You need to find out what works best for you.

Now, say you do an exercise for 10 sets of 10 reps to failure with a 2-minute rest time. That's a total of 100 reps with 20 minutes of rest. That is a tough workout and for reps 8, 9, and 10 on most of the sets, especially the later sets, those will be extremely difficult.

In fact, you probably won't be able to complete that workout with the same weight. You'll have to drop the weight just to maintain doing 10 reps for each set.

In the whole scheme of things, these types of workouts simply won't work over the long term. Your progress will stall out and plateau because this is too hard on your Nervous System and muscles. Intensity is good, but not when it's done incorrectly (and too often) like in that example.

Here's a better way: With the 10 sets of 10 reps with two minutes rest (you'll need a longer rest time with higher reps), you end up doing 100 reps with a total of 20 minutes of rest time.

Note: Most people think they need longer rest times with lower reps and heavier weights because higher reps and lighter weights are "easier." That is simply *wrong*. The weight may be easier, but it's not easier on your Nervous System. Remember, this method is all about the Nervous System.

So what you'd do instead of the 10 by 10 with a 2-minute rest time is this:

20 sets of 5 reps with 30 second rest times.

Guess what happens then?

You end up doing the same 100 reps, but you do it with just 10 minutes of rest times. Read that again! It's very important to clearly see what just happened there.

And also, you do it all with the same weight since all the sets will be *easy*. You won't struggle at all. Not only that, you could do the same workout the next day because your muscles and Nervous System are fine. Your muscles are also fresh.

If you don't believe me, try it with basically any exercise.

Pick an exercise and weight and do it 10 sets of 10 reps with a two-minute rest time between sets. Make sure the weight is heavy enough so that you'd fail on your 11th rep. A week later, pick the same exercise and weight and do it for 20 sets of 5 reps with a 30-second rest time between sets.

You'll feel better during the second workout compared to the first workout. The second workout will be easier to do. You'll be able to do the second workout in about half the time of the first workout (increasing your exercise density... the same or more exercise done in less time). How does that not improve your body!

You'll be able to maintain the same weight throughout every set and every rep of the second workout. You won't be able to maintain the same weight for every set and every rep during the first workout.

The next day you'll feel fine after the second workout. Plus, you'll be able to do all of it again. With the first workout, nope, you would not be able to do it again so quickly because you exhausted your Nervous System (this overrides your muscles; even if your muscles are NOT exhausted and are fine).

The bottom line is you'll be able to do more volume and more total weight in less time with the Effortless Exercising Method no matter what exercises you choose to use it with. You'll be able to do all that within the workout. Think of the possibilities with the exercises you're currently doing.

But just as important, you can do these workouts more often (in less total time each week), which leads to even more volume which leads to more toning and more weight loss.

Consider the following.

Let's say you and a friend had the same body and the same goals. If you did the Effortless Exercise Method and your friend did the traditional way of exercising using reps to failure (and cardio to exhaustion), your progress would be light years ahead of her progress.

A year later she won't even be close. You'll be far more toned and look a lot better... and feel better.

Main Concept #4: H.F.I.

Consider another vital formula from the Effortless Exercising Method for Women:

Specificity + Frequent Practice = Superior Performance

In other words, you want High Frequency and Intensity (H.F.I).

If you play sports or have kids who play sports, use that formula to become or help your child become a superior athlete. Sure, there's a *little* more to it than that, but that's the basic formula and the approach works wonders.

If you want to get good at pushups, you specifically do a lot of pushups. If you want to get good at pull-ups, you specifically do a lot of pull-ups.

It's actually pretty simple.

Sure, you can help increase the amount of pushups and pull-ups you do by doing other things. But that would be an inefficient way to master the two exercises. Want to do more pull-ups or whatever exercise... then do that specific exercise, often.

Drawbacks

The two main drawbacks to high frequency training of an exercise using typical workout methods are muscular fatigue and burning out your central nervous system (CNS). Because of those two things, you won't be able to train often. Your body needs time to recover to perform at a high level.

That's where short rests, low reps, and lots of sets come in.

Higher reps to muscular failure absolutely destroy your CNS recovery[10] infinitely more than low reps not to failure. However, you condition your body to get more toned and lose fat by being able to handle more and more volume without burning out your CNS and destroying your muscles' ability to recover.

Low reps (without being physically tired doing them) work perfectly to imprint the movement into your CNS for gains not only in the movement, but also in your whole body. This results in a more efficient CNS results in mind-muscle connection that leads to improved gains.

The gains will lead to far more toning in your muscles.

By not going to failure, you can increase the volume of sets that you do while you're fresh. The short rest times help release growth hormone (GH)[11] during your workout. Long rest times don't do that. You can use longer rest times than what I outline if you want, but short rest times simply work better since you aren't going to failure during any sets.

It's nice to know, isn't it, that you'll still be fresh even with a 30 second or less rest between sets. But, if you're not ready to do another set in 30 to 45 seconds, then you did too many reps the previous set or sets.

Remember that. If you don't feel fresh for another set in 30-45 seconds, you did too much the previous set and you need to cut it back.

Not only do you save time working out with shorter rest times, you also get the added benefit of a GH release during your workout. The great thing about shorter rest times is that is where you imprint intensity into your workouts... SAFELY (for your Nervous System).

Please get it out of your head that you have to do as many reps as possible until you can't do any more. That will hurt your recovery which forces you to workout less which will lead to doing less total volume which leads to slow or no progress. I'm harping on this, but I can't stress it enough.

Instead of thinking about doing as many reps per set, think in terms of doing a certain amount of total reps for the workout.

Who cares how many sets it takes to do them all?

In the other parts of this book I've given you outlines of how many reps you should do in order to get a stronger and toned.

Once you can do all those reps as outlined, then your next progression is simply to do all those reps in a shorter time by lowering the rest time between sets or increasing the amount of sets you do. Or do both.

If you lower the rest times, it'll help more for getting toned and losing fat.

Note: I sometimes hear women tell me they want to get toned but not necessarily "stronger." It's difficult to separate the two. If you improve your muscular tone you get stronger.

If you increase the amount of sets, it'll help more for gaining muscle tone. You can also carefully increase the amount of reps per set.

But this is the most important thing: Be careful because you can't come close to muscular failure during any set since you need to keep your muscles and CNS fresh.

For superior performance, you need to perform while you're fresh. If your muscles along with your CNS are exhausted, then you won't have superior performance during practice or competition. If your muscles and CNS are constantly fried throughout the week, you won't be able to practice enough to become a superior athlete or performer in the first place (unless of course you're gifted).

It's that simple.

And that is true for people trying to get stronger too. It doesn't matter if you want to be a superior athlete or not.

Frequency and Effectiveness

Now one thing I want to clear up. High frequency by itself isn't anything special. For example, you might walk a lot, but somehow this frequency of walking doesn't make your legs bigger or stronger or even more toned.

Why is that?

It's because walking isn't very intense. Frequency needs to be teamed up with intensity. Once an exercise becomes too easy for you, you need to graduate to another exercise or figure out a way to make that exercise more intense.

Think of the following:

- Are people who walk a lot big and strong, generally speaking? No.

- Are people who jog a lot big and strong, generally speaking? No.

- Are people who sprint often big and strong, generally speaking? Yes!

The Difference

Sprinting is intense, but walking and jogging aren't intense. So it doesn't matter how often you do something that isn't intense enough to elicit adaptation from your body. There is a balancing act between intensity and recovery.

The best way to use intensity to reach your body goals is within the framework of the Effortless Exercise Method, which allows for a faster recovery rate for your body.

Now, maybe your goal isn't to become as strong as possible.

Maybe you just want to stay in shape. For many of us, that's great because we have children and our lives to fill all the time we have. Simply lower the intensity level of what you're doing. You're still building neurological efficiency into your body and muscles, but you're not building it in a way to elicit a lot more strength.

> **Note:** Let me rephrase that so we're clear. First, I'm just using walking and jogging and sprinting as examples to getting bigger and stronger. You may as well not want to get bigger muscles. That's fine. These principles work just as well for losing weight and toning up. I want to reiterate again... don't be afraid that by using these principles you'll get big "guy" muscles. Guys have genetics and extra testosterone that help them develop those big muscles. Most women don't. So you won't get big muscles when

37

trying to lose weight and tone up.

Just keep this in mind: Training to muscular failure with high reps results in *no long-term progress*.[12]

Muscle Recovery

There's one other related issue we need to discuss.

It's a myth that it takes your muscles two to four days to recover and repair. The reason why most people think that is because they train wrong. They're training to failure too often (maybe every set). They do as many repetitions as possible until they can't do any more for the set.

Again, females aren't as prone to this as men but I've seen enough that I must still warn you about it.

Beating up your body may lead to gains and adaptations early on, but over the long-term your body will tap out and not go along for that ride. And this is why they can't progress and will plateau out quickly and be stuck there for maybe years.

They can't get in the volume of work they need (in a state of freshness for the Nervous System) to stimulate strength and growth because the way they're training forces them to train each muscle group only once or twice a week.

Bulgarian Olympic lifters are some of the strongest people in the world.[13] They train up to 28 times a week. Yes, 28 times! Sure, you don't want to be an Olympic lifter, but I use this example to demonstrate that recovery times are too often misunderstood.

How can those guys train so often and still be some of the strongest people in the world? Simple (and now obvious): They don't train to failure.

They lift heavy, but they don't lift their maximum weight. They also don't lift until they can't lift the weight again. They cut their sets short and do short workouts to keep their bodies fresh and their recovery minimal.

Understand this...

Never destroy yourself doing a set (with weights, bodyweight, or cardio). Don't go all out on a set. You need intensity, so you need the set to be kind of hard, but don't push yourself too much. Instead let the set be part of a bigger picture. Let the accumulated volume of your sets take care of your body improvements.

By the way, if you find that you want to gain more strength but minimize any possible muscle gains from forming, just increase your rest times. The reason for this is because longer rest times do two things: they lower and also limit the release of growth hormone (GH) during your workouts. Since growth hormone is a key hormone for gaining muscle, you're then reducing your ability to gain muscle.

Men must monitor this more than women, but for those who do work out a lot, keep an eye on this.

Keep in mind, too, that longer rest times mean less total workout volume overall in a given timeframe. Since there is less stimulation of your muscles, they have less reason to grow. So always keep that in mind.

You can use the Effortless Exercise Method to gain both strength and toned muscles or lose weight by adjusting how you work it. It's up to you how you use these concepts and this method.

Easy Breezy

Anyway, the final thought for this section is to remember that everything about the Effortless Exercise Method revolves around each set being easy. Easy, but with intensity. The easiness comes from you stopping the set short before it becomes hard. The intensity comes from the short rest times between sets.

The accumulated amount of work you do from all these easy sets combined with your ability to do them more often will easily surpass any results you get from doing fewer, harder sets that wipe you out.

Fortunately, a simple test tells you if you were successful or not: If your mind doesn't feel energized after you finished a workout, then you did something wrong.

4
MINI-WORKOUTS

If you're extremely busy, trying to plan and fit in a workout sucks. I'm about to give you a new way at looking at exercise.

You think you need to do 30 or more minutes or it's pointless to work out. So what ends up happening is you skip a lot of workouts just because it's too inconvenient and hard to find the time to do them.

These missed workouts add up.

They stall your progress. They sap your motivation. And eventually you may just throw up your arms in the air and give up on the whole exercise thing. Instead, you think, you'll just focus on doing some extreme diet, minus the working out.

You don't need long, 30 or more minute workouts to lose weight and tone up. You certainly don't need to do a lot of jogging. You can use mini-workouts. The idea is simple. Fit in your exercise whenever and wherever you have one to five minutes of free time.

What happens when you do this is you get in a lot of volume (sets) each day by doing a set here and there throughout the day.

Because I was and am so busy myself, I developed this way of working out because I was missing too many workouts. Everyone, no matter how busy, can spare 1 to 5 minutes of time 5 to 20 times a day, here and there.

You can to.

At first you'll need to plan these mini-workouts, but soon they'll become an ingrained habit that you do without even having to think about doing them.

Perhaps the biggest benefit to doing a bunch of mini-workouts daily (instead of a long workout) is the multiple times you give a kick to your metabolism to speed up. Each time you do a mini-workout, you're training your metabolism to work at a faster speed.

Do this often enough and eventually your metabolism will take those temporary boosts in speed and make them permanent. That is where things really take off for real and long term fat loss. A faster metabolism causes you to burn more calories every single minute of the day!

TV Commercials Helped Me!

The key is to develop these mini-workouts into a habit or you may forget to do them. What's worked best for me is to do these mini-workouts during TV commercials. The typical TV show today has 2 to 3 minutes of commercials about 8 times an hour. So, that's about 20 minutes an hour of "free" time (or wasted time) for exercise.

So, this is simple.

I'm telling you to watch at least an hour of TV a day. It's okay. I give you permission. *But* during those commercials, I want you to exercise. Combine watching TV with getting a healthier, better, sexier body.

You never need to find separate time to work out. Include your workouts during TV time (or while you're on the computer... or whenever). I will include exercises you can do during TV commercials shortly.

You don't *have* to focus solely on doing mini-workouts during TV commercials.

You can do these mini-workouts at work, during your lunch hour, or pretty much whenever. Sometimes I do them while I'm cooking. Sometimes I do them when I come out of the bathroom (okay, maybe that was too much information).

The only limit is your own creativity as to when you do them. Figure out what works best for you and make sure to do *a lot* of these mini-workouts throughout each day.

By doing this, you can easily fit in 30 to 60 (or more) minutes of working out daily in segments of 1 to 5 minutes at a time.

5
THE 4-MINUTE WORKOUT

I want you to try Tabata-based jumping jacks.

I know, you probably think jumping jacks are a joke. I did too. But that's because there are a few key things you weren't doing when you did jumping jacks. If you use the proper workout protocol and you seriously put effort into them, jumping jacks will beat you down (in a good way).

Tabata is a form of interval training.[14] Tabata requires just four minutes of your time. But it's an extremely intense four minutes, even with simple exercises. It becomes 20 seconds of exercise followed by 10 seconds of rest. You will keep repeating that for a total of four minutes.

> **Note:** You need to be *precise* with those times for this to be effective. Too many people turn 10-second rests into 20 to 30 second rests. You may need slightly longer rest times at first, but eventually you need to use the 20-10 protocol.

This exercise format is really intense and you can use it for a whole bunch of other exercises too. I recommend that you do this twice a week to change things up from the other exercises. This means it will take you just 8 minutes of your time for the whole week.

Note: This routine is an exception to the Effortless Exercising principles talked about previously. As long as you do this just twice a week, you will be fine and won't cause any exhaustion problems for your Nervous System.

The whole concept is named after Dr. Tabata who discovered that this type of interval training produces much better fat loss results than aerobic training. It's not even a close comparison. In fact, *four minutes doing the Tabata interval is equal to doing 45 minutes of normal cardio training!*

You may want to read that again because it's profound and revolutionary.

The four minutes of doing Tabata intervals may feel like the longest four minutes of your life too, but it will be worth it.

Here's how you do them.

You can do almost any exercise for Tabata intervals, but in this case, I recommend power jumping jacks. You should do the jumping jacks as fast as possible for 20 seconds non-stop. Then you rest 10 seconds. You will repeat them doing as many power jumping jacks as possible for another 20 seconds and resting 10 seconds.

Keep repeating that sequence until the four minutes are over (actually 3 minutes and 50 seconds). You'll do 8 total sets of the 20-10 sequence. Try to be as accurate as possible with your timing. If you have a stopwatch feature on your watch or phone, use that. Or if you have a clock with a moving hand, do this while watching the clock. I personally use a Gymboss timer.

Just remember the key: Do the jumping jacks as fast as possible. Don't do them slowly! This isn't meant to be a casual exercise. You're going to take an easy exercise like jumping jacks and make it hard and effective for fat loss.

Just in case you want to see how to do jumping jacks, here is a quick video I found through a Google search:

http://www.youtube.com/watch?v=dmYwZH_BNd0

Note that the video's star did not do the jumping jacks explosively or as fast as possible. You however will. That is the key to making jumping jacks effective. You will do them explosively and as fast as possible. I can't stress that enough. By doing that and using the Tabata Protocol, you'll get quite the mini-workout for fat loss.

1-Minute Protocol

Use the same Tabata protocols to run in place. But instead of four minutes, just do it for one minute.

Here's the 1-minute protocol:

1. 25 seconds of running in place as fast as you can

2. 15 seconds of rest

3. 20 seconds of running in place as fast as you can

That's it. It takes just one minute. You can run during TV commercials. You don't need to set aside huge chunks of time to work out. Make your workouts fit into your busy schedule.

If you can do this 1-minute Tabata version 3 to 5 times each day, you'll get really good fat loss results. But the key is to really put in the effort when you're running. Move your legs and arms as fast as possible. (This is by no means effortless, but when you do them in short bursts like this you won't have any problem with your Nervous System when not following the Effortless Exercise Method principles.)

If you don't give it 100% effort, you won't get the great results that I'm promising you. Don't worry about how fast you're going. You can go slowly if you need to, especially at first. Just worry about your effort and intent to do it fast.

It may be slow for other people, but if it's fast for you, then you'll lose a bunch of fat.

Another "Intense" Way to do Cardio

HIIT stands for *High Intensity Interval Training*.[15] If the thought of aerobic movement such as running for hours on end sounds like a nightmare to you, you're going to like HIIT a lot.

This is one of the fastest ways to burn fat off your body when it comes to cardio. Long drawn out jogging is an inefficient way to try and lose weight. It actually eats away at your muscles. The result can be horribly bad because when you lose muscle mass, you force your body to slow your metabolic rate.

The way to do cardio is to vary the intensity by going from really easy up to really intense and then repeat that. As an example, say you are on the elliptical or stairstepper.

You'll want to do 10 to 15 seconds of all out intensity... as hard as you can go cardio. Then follow that by doing 30 to 45 seconds of easy cardio. And keep repeating that for a total of 6 minute "sets." So out of a total of 6 minutes, about 4 and 1/2 minutes are easy.

But that other minute and a half is extremely intense!

Note: The HITT method is sort of an exception to the effortless exercise principles even though most of the exercise time during HITT is actually easy.

After six minutes get off and drink some water. Rest 3 to 5 minutes. Then get back on and do again.

You can repeat this for a total of 24 to 30 minutes on the machine. Doing this is perfect for gym workouts. That's it.

And you can practice this with running outdoors too.

Run hard for 10 to 15 seconds and then walk for 45 to 50 seconds. Keep repeating that for ten minutes. Trust me. Ten minutes is all you'll need if you did it. Forget long, drawn-out jogging!

> **Note**: Don't do this sprinting on a treadmill since the sudden changes of speed is hard on your legs. Plus, the fast-and-slow-and-fast progressions aren't usually practical on a treadmill.

What is truly great about this type of cardio is that not only do you burn a lot of fat, but you also burn fat *at an accelerated rate* for 18 to 36 hours *after* this short-but-intense workout... while you're NOT working out. Your metabolism gets a fat burning jolt for up to a day and a half after doing it.

That is the key that makes this one of the most efficient ways to burn fat from exercising.

If you're going to do cardio, consider using High Intensity Intervals so you get the accelerated rate of fat burning for 18+ hours after the workout. Your body becomes a fat burning machine for the whole day. It's programmed into being in hyper fat burning mode.

6
THE EXERCISES

Here are some exercise suggestions. You'll see that these are just suggestions. You can use the Effortless Exercise principles, Tabata, and HIIT with whatever exercises you want.

You don't need to strictly limit yourself to the following exercises. For the most part, the principles are more important than the exercises. Do what you can and do what you want.

Some of the exercises you might not be able to do or might not have the equipment to do. That's fine. Just do something else. I'm giving you some simple outlines and exercises to consider, but remember, you're free to go in whatever direction you want. You're in control of this journey. Just pick and choose.

Jumping A Special Way

Jumping on a mini-trampoline is not only a great exercise, but it's good for your cells. You can get a mini-trampoline (called a *rebounder*) at Walmart for about $25 to $30 (if you're not in North America, do a search on the internet on where you can get it).

Note: Rebounders do wonders for your immune

system![16]

The rebounder is great to jump on for two minutes here and there. Those two minutes of jumping add up. As with so many other exercises, a great time to use this is during commercials while you're watching TV. So when you watch TV, do so with a mini-trampoline in front of you!

During each commercial, I want you to jump on the mini-trampoline. At the end of an hour, you would have jumped on the trampoline for 15 to 20 minutes. Don't use the excuse that you don't have time to do this. And if you don't watch TV, I'm sure you can still find a couple of minutes here and there throughout the day to jump on the mini-trampoline at home (before eating is a good time to do it for a couple minutes).

Besides during commercials, I also jump on the mini-trampoline before and after going to the bathroom (too much information again?), while I'm cooking, and after I put laundry in the washing machine. That's just my routine.

If you're watching your kids, you can do it with them. Take turns. They love it!

Come on... don't think of lame excuses on why you can't do this. It's simple, your kids would like it, and it can be done in your home anytime you feel like it. Plus the rebounder is small and you can leave it in your living room.

This is an exercise that I do almost *every day*! It's convenient, but it's also great for your cells. Doing this helps maintain a "youthfulness" to your cells due to its effects on improving the lymphatic system and its circulation throughout your body.

The mini-trampoline helps to allow you to avoid going to the gym... saving the $40+ a month for a gym membership. It also saves me hours of driving to and from the gym. It also saves my cells and helps me to become younger at the "cellular level" because of my improved lymphatic system.

Circular Motions

If you have flabby arms that annoy you, this is one of the best things you can do to tone them up. This exercise won't help with weight loss, but it's great for the localized effect of toning your arms.

Put your arms out like airplane wings so they are at shoulder level.

Then start moving them in small circles… just moving your arms a few inches in these circles.

Now, you won't get quick toning results on your arms from this alone. But these arm circles definitely help a lot. Combined with dieting and cardio exercises, you will lose a lot of the jiggly arm flab.

I suggest you do these for 1 minute at a time. If possible, do for a total of 5 minutes a day if you want to focus on toning your arms.

If you don't have much arm flab, then you can probably skip these and just focus on dieting and cardio to tone up your arms without you specifically doing any arm exercises.

This Kind of Squatting Is Ladylike!

The bodyweight squat is another great exercise you can do at home or anywhere you find yourself. The bodyweight squat is great for your butt and legs.

The deeper you squat down, the more the squat tightens and firms your butt.

To begin, figure out how many you can do in one set.

Initially, just do as many as possible until you can't do anymore. You'll need to find that limit in order to implement the effortless exercise principle.

As an example, say you can do 20 total bodyweight squats for a set until you can't do anymore. What you'll want to do is sets of ten squats in order to manage your fatigue and allow you to do more sets with shorter rest times.

Doing this achieves all the goals of the Effortless Exercise plan.

7

A PREMIER 5-MINUTE MIRACLE EXERCISE THAT SAYS "NO" TO THE STAIRSTEPPER AND "YES" TO FAT LOSS

If I could rank one of the top fat-loss exercises in existence, this may be it. Stair Runs-Walks. It fits all our criteria of being simple, convenient, not requiring expensive equipment, and the regimen is not time intensive.

This turns things from "Running Sucks" to "Running is Great."

And guess what the best part is? This fat-loss exercise will not only help your overall fitness and reduce your fat, it helps you develop a firm butt too!

The Only Requirement

Obviously, no exercise named *Stair Runs-Walks* is going to be possible without some stairs somewhere. Certainly you should not buy or rent something like a Stairmaster. That is *way* over the top and wastes your time, money, and space... and a stair-stepper would hurt your results anyway. All you need are some sturdy stairs at home. If you have those, you're ready to roll and everything will be totally convenient.

If you don't have inside stairs, do you possibly have some outside stairs or a building with stairs nearby?

What Not to Do

Yes, I know you want the specifics. But humor me because before going further it's critical that I describe what *not* to do before I describe what you *should* do.

> **Note:** I caution you to *not* go out and try this exercise at its fullest right away.

Unless you're in good condition already and actively exercise a lot, you probably won't be able to handle this workout right away. That is just fine. It is best to build up to it.

But as the song goes, don't worry, be happy!

The good news is this: Your results from this exercise will be so quick that even if it takes you two weeks to begin doing the exercise exactly as outlined, you're still *way* ahead of everyone else.

The Routine

The plan for *Stair Runs-Walks* is simple. Here is what you do:

1. Run up one to three flights of stairs.

2. When you get to the top, walk back down the stairs.

3. When you get back to the bottom of the stairs, run back up them.

4. Repeat as many times as possible for five minutes *without* stopping.

A big part of the reason why this is so efficient at burning off body fat is because you are always moving.

You do get a rest on the walks down the stairs, but it's an active rest. It is not a passive rest.

Note: Have you watched Olympic runners? After an agonizing run, whether sprinting or long-distance, the runners hit the finish line and in spite of the fact they are exhausted they do not lie down. Instead they *walk!* You'd think the last thing they want to do is keep moving but a heavy-breathing slow walk *is* how they recover. The human body seems to want to recover from an exhaustive run by walking and moving, albeit at a much slower pace.[17]

Added Bonus Benefits

These between-run walks give you an added bonus benefit. You don't get a complete rest before you have to run up the stairs again. You will find that you will need to take a lot of deep breaths. You will consume oxygen heavily.

About the deep breaths... those add to your fat-burning. The walks between each stair run turn you into a fat-burning machine!

"Why is that?" you ask? It's science, but simple science. For your body to burn off fat and use that fat for energy, your body must combine your fat with oxygen to release that fat effectively and efficiently. The more oxygen you breathe into your lungs and, therefore, ultimately into your bloodstream, the more body fat you will burn.

Note: Consider this: If you skipped exercising completely and only performed several deep breathing exercises throughout the day, you would increase your body's fat loss by the deep breathing alone. It won't be nearly as effective as breathing while exercising, but it'll still burn more body fat than if you do not exercise. That oxygen is a nice, effective fat-burning agent. And given that this exercise requires only *five minutes*, and that's once you work up *to* five minutes, you just have no excuse not to spend those five minutes on the stairs *and* getting that healthy fat-burning oxygen.

Remember, even if your body begins getting used to the Stair Runs-Walks and can get through the first two or three minutes without breathing heavily, I encourage you to consciously perform a deep breathing pattern on the walks to maximize your fat loss.

Just don't use deep breathing alone as a substitute for the Stair Runs-Walks.

The Stair Run-Walks exercise has additional fat-loss benefits. Not only does the deep breathing become far heavier and unforced as you get into the exercise's rhythm, but also the actual movement you perform helps you a great deal too.

Obvious you don't move when you're doing deep breathing without exercise. And perhaps most important, deep breathing alone won't help you develop a firm butt like the way this exercise will.

The bottom line is that body fat needs a lot of oxygen present in order to burn itself off and be released. Most people only shallow breathe, they rarely exercise, and they usually breathe polluted air. We don't get as much oxygen as we should into our cells. Think back 100 years when most families lived on a farm or in a country environment.

The clean outside air combined with their labor made them lean naturally.

With modern times, we get the good with the bad. With our tablet computers and office jobs we get thicker thighs and hipper hips. Ugh! It's a good thing we can do something about those to help make up for what we give up for modern living.

ATP

The actual fat burning process where energy is created and released depends on something called *adenosine triphosphate* or *ATP* for short.[18] By oxygenating your body's cells through the exercise-induced deep breathing, your body produces an environment that encourages the production of ATP. With more ATP you get more fat burning.

And that's the boring science behind it. Fortunately we don't have to be scientists to have thinner thighs and waistlines.

On Getting Started

The first thing you need to do is test yourself on one to three flights of stairs.

> **Note:** By the way, your goal should be to run up the stairs in the range of five to fifteen seconds or so. One flight of stairs isn't necessarily worse than 3 flights depending on how long it takes you.

Just choose what works best for you and put in the effort.

Once you know how in-shape you are, you can decide how hard you will seriously try to do the full five minutes of running up the stairs and walking down the stairs. Non-stop.

How you do this is up to you.

I strongly encourage you to take it slowly for the first one to two weeks if you're not very athletic. This gives your body a chance to build up, extend your abilities, and to make sure you don't become overly sore or hurt. Becoming too sore too soon will discourage you and you won't want to continue this waist-reducing routine.

What I'd like for you to do for the first day is spend only one minute running up the stairs and walking down them. Don't stop during that one minute. Repeat this sequence five separate times during the day for a total of 5 minutes.

Mix it up at first. Listen to your body to decide what will challenge you without exerting you.

For example, you could spend one full minute doing the Runs-Walks, stop and rest one full minute, and so on until you've completed the full five minutes of Stair Run-Walks. Or, you can do one minute here and there throughout the day... even if you do so several hours apart.

It's all up to you.

Bumping it Up

Once you feel you that you have fully mastered those one-minute Stair Runs-Walks, you're ready to do a full two minutes of non-stop Stair Runs-Walks.

Then, once you've mastered that, bump up to doing them for three minutes, again non-stop. Keep going to four minutes non-stop, and then finally you'll be doing it for the full five minutes non-stop.

> **Note:** When you first read about the Stair Runs-Walks, you may be fooled into thinking that five minutes isn't much at all. Trust me, you will find out the first time you begin this exercise that five minutes *at first* is like an eternity.

For the average person, moving up to the five-minute level will take somewhere between one to three weeks. If you're somewhat athletic and in shape when you begin, then the full five minutes of non-stop Stair Runs-Walks should take you a week or less.

Whatever you do, do not concede the race before you even begin it! Don't feel that you have to be able to do the Stair Runs-Walks for five minutes, non-stop, immediately.

Most people can't.

Once you master the top level, stay with it and don't go more than the five minutes. You'll reach a point of diminishing returns beyond that due to what we mentioned earlier about the Nervous System being overtaxed.

Now, to be clear this is not an "effortless" exercise.

You will definitely feel the effort. This directly contradicts the Effortless Exercise Method principles. I want to stress this again so that you're not confused. Since the time amounts to 5 minutes or less, you can break the Effortless Exercise Method principles and get great results due to how limited the time is (5 minutes or less) which isn't enough time for the intensity to cause a "frying" of your Nervous System.

After doing the Stair Runs-walks for five minutes non-stop, five days a week, for two weeks, you will almost certainly have lost at least five pounds of fat from this one exercise alone.

And keep this in mind: the time it has taken you to read just this far into *Running Sucks* is *far* more time than you'll use up doing Stair Runs-Walks over several days' time! In other words, those five pounds are coming off not because you have built up to become a marathon runner, but only because you've built up to five minutes!

And for many of you, you're doing this inside your own home! Running was never as good as this, or as effective!

An Alternative

In spite of how easy the Stair Runs-Walks sound when you first read about them, some people find them too challenging. I want to offer an alternative just in case you're unable to do the running part of these Stair Runs-Walks.

Almost anybody can do this alternative routine. And if you're one who needs to begin here, you may find that you work up to the actual Stair Runs-Walks that I described above.

The downside to the alternative, though, is that you'll need to do it for 20 minutes a day, six days a week, for two weeks to get the same results as the five minutes of unmodified Stair Runs-Walks just five days a week. (The oxygen that the actual Stair Runs-Walks infuses into your system is a major helper.)

The alternative is simply walking up and down one to three flights of stairs, non-stop, for 20 minutes each day.

Since you'll need to do this for six days a week; that's a total of two hours of exercise time for the week. It reduces the time benefit of the Stair Runs-Walks, but it's something that almost anybody can do and it does help anyone, who does them, burn off fat.

Really, 20 minutes daily isn't much, especially if you have stairs conveniently located in your home. Make sure that you have a good audio book or music to listen to and the 20 minutes will fly by. Still, 20 minutes a day adding up to two hours a week is obviously way more time than the daily five minutes a day that requires only 25 total minutes each week.

Still, there's nothing wrong with starting with the alternative if you need to.

You may find that your joints take the alternative better and stick with it. As we age, being able to run even on a flat surface gets trickier. Do whatever *you* need to do. I just wanted to add this easier alternative since not everyone can run up stairs. Either way, get ready to lose a lot of fat really fast.

The bottom line is this: go find some stairs and start running and walking on them. A stair-stepper is not as effective. Use REAL stairs.

8
BUMPING UP YOUR GAME

So many other ways exist to burn your fat, or improve your body, easily without running that we'd better get to them.

Build a Better Butt!

Isometric Butt Squeezes are simple and you can do them standing up or lying down on your stomach.

Just squeeze your butt together using your gluteus muscles. Squeeze as hard as you can for one to ten seconds. Repeat for at least five minutes a day to tone and firm your butt.

You can "squeeze" this in anytime. You don't need to do the whole five minutes all at once.

I personally do these while lying down and watching TV (there I go again with too much information shared).

Yes, these sound too good to be true. They are truly effortless and a great way to firm your butt.

The Best all-Around At-Home Exercise... *Period!*

I'm going to go a little deeper here because this exercise deserves the coverage.

Burpees are becoming known far and wide, but sadly the Burpee has been considered a "guys" exercise. That is unfair because women can and should do Burpees if their goal is to lose fat as fast as possible while toning up their whole body.

The Burpee is a bodyweight movement. You don't even need stairs as you do with the Stairs Runs-Walks exercise. You can do Burpees at home and all you need is a little bit of open space.

The Routine

Here's how to do Burpees:

1. Begin in a squat position with your hands on the floor in front of you. Don't plant your feet at too wide of angles outward from your centerline. Keep your feet pointed fairly straight.

2. Kick your feet back while you go down into a pushup.

3. As you're pushing up with the quick pushup, return your feet into your previous squat position.

4. Jump up as high as you can from the squat position. Congratulations! This is a Burpee!

5. Keep repeating the Burpees, doing them as fast as possible.

Now, doing Burpees will require that you *aren't* totally out of shape. If you cannot do them, slow down as much as you need to and build up over time. You know how they say, "No pain, no gain"? This is so true of Burpees. In the exercise community there is almost a full consensus that the Burpee is the best fat-burning exercise one can do without equipment.

To illustrate the proper way to do Burpees, it's best that you see them in action. Here's a web page with a picture of

Burpees:

http://myfitnesshut.blogspot.com/2010/11/burpees-burn-fat.html

Perhaps even more helpful, here is a video of Burpees being performed properly: http://www.youtube.com/watch?v=c_Dq_NCzj8M

Your personal goal for Burpees should be for you to find out how many you can do in 1 set where you go to failure and can't do anymore. Once you know that, apply the Effortless Exercise Method principles (sets, reps, rest times, etc.) and do at most half the reps of your maximum set while doing a lot of sets.

This maximizes fat loss while keeping your Nervous System fresh... allowing you to do this daily.

As an example, say you can do a total of 10 Burpees and no more in a set. Then you do a lot of sets of 4-5 Burpees with short rest times. As this gets easier for you, you can increase the amount of reps per set to 5-6, and so on (because your capacity to do more Burpees in a set to failure increases).

You can also increase the amount of sets. In addition, you can lower the amount of time you rest between sets. Just follow the Effortless Exercises Method principles and make sure each set is fairly simple while you build up the volume. If you can eventually build up to 100 Burpees a day, you probably won't even need to do any other exercises.

You'll see why!

Scheduling Them

It might not surprise you that, if nothing else, I encourage you to do Burpees during TV commercials.

Instead of purely using my Effortless Exercise

principles, you can do as many Burpees as you can in one minute. Then stop and wait for the next commercial. Then do as many Burpees as you can in one minute. But again, you can also use my Effortless Exercise principles for Burpees during commercials as well.

Your choice. I'm just giving you a few different options.

You should keep doing Burpees for a total of five commercials and five total minutes.

This is the easiest way I've found to add Burpees into your schedule every day. If you're able to combine five minutes of Burpees and five minutes of Stair Runs-Walks each day for five days a week, your body really has no choice but to burn off a lot of fat.

> **Note:** Obviously, the five days that make the most sense are the five weekdays. Skipping days here and there makes losing count too easy, enables you to not get a full five days in every seven-day period, and ultimately can hinder you enough to make you quit before the fat loss is finished.

Rolling Away Cellulite

If you have cellulite[19] on your butt and or legs, using a foam roller is one of the best ways to help diminish and reduce it.

Full Disclosure: This is not a miracle. This won't totally get rid of your cellulite. This does take time to see results. Still, I won't waste your time so understand that foam rolling is a great and easy thing to do to make a dent on the dreaded cellulite.

A foam roller is a firm foam log that's about 6 inches in diameter. Here's a picture of one.

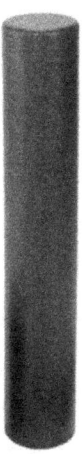

Get a 6-inch by 36-inch foam roller. If you're not in the USA, do a Google search for "foam rollers" or go to your local department store's sporting goods section. Here is the link to one at Amazon:

http://www.amazon.com/Fit-36-Inch-Hi-Density-Foam-Roller/dp/B0028KDC82

Use the foam roller against your cellulite areas by rolling on it with your weight. It acts like a massage for the area you're rolling on. The foam roller helps flush your tissues and improve the circulation of lymph and blood to your cellulite areas.

The lack of good blood flow along with your lymph nodes getting clogged up often contributes to the formation of cellulite.

That is why "massaging out" your cellulite areas with a foam roller will reduce the appearance of the cellulite. Yes, it takes time. Be patient. After all, in six months, you'll be six months older whether you use the roller or not. Why not be six months older with better-looking thighs?

Note: The foam roller can also be used as a rehab aid for joints and muscle pain.

9
THREE EXERCISES FOR THAT CURVY, FEMININE HOURGLASS FIGURE

If you want to have a body that is like an hourglass, nice and curvy, while still looking skinny, I have 3 specific exercises you should do to help accentuate your curves.

For an hourglass figure, you need to have toned and slightly wide shoulders. But don't worry. You won't get "guy shoulders." Understand that you need wider and better-toned shoulders to help give the illusion of your waist being smaller. It's the contrast between them that helps make your waist look smaller.

You'll also need to work on making your waist and love handles smaller.

Finally, you'll need to develop your outer thighs. Why your outer thighs? Because with wider shoulders, a smaller waist, and outer thighs that are slightly bigger and toned, you create an hourglass figure. Your outer thighs will also contrast with your thinner waist.

The Three Exercises

The first exercise is the bodyweight squat that I listed

above already. The key to doing the bodyweight squat to build the outer thighs and help you create the illusion of a better hourglass figure is to keep your feet close to each other.

I suggest you do *bodyweight squats* with your feet about 6 inches apart. Do the bodyweight squats as listed above.

Don't worry about building up your thighs a little (if your goal is to have an hourglass figure). Remember, the goal is to make your waist look smaller while also making you look more curvy and feminine. You won't get big "guy" legs from bodyweight squats. You're basically toning your thighs, but with emphasis on the outer thighs.

Banding Apart

The second exercise you should master is called *band pullaparts*.

Band pullaparts help you tone the outside of your shoulders to make them slightly wider. A side benefit is that these are also great for shoulder health.

You'll need a mini-band or a light band to do these. These only cost a few dollars (if you're not in the USA, again, just do a Google search for them or go to a sporting goods store.

Here's the EFS Pro Short Mini Band, the one I bought due to its high quality:

http://www.flexcart.com/members/elitefts/default.asp?m=PD&cid=114&pid=3254

Please note that weightlifters also use bands, but they use them for different reasons and for different exercises. So get that band or a band similar to the one I got, shown here:

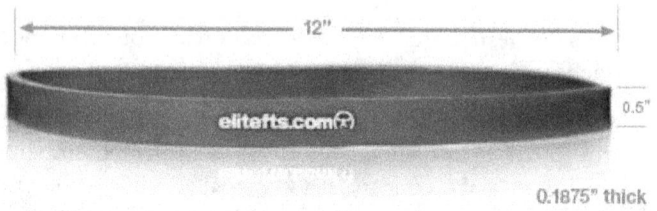

12"

0.5"

0.1875" thick

Ok, you have the band.

Now, while standing up with your arms straight out in front of you at shoulder level, hook each of your thumbs into each side of the band. Now pull the band apart with your thumbs.

Because of the tension of the band, you'll only be able to stretch it out six to twelve inches. That's all you need.

Do at least 100 of these a day. Each time you pull the band apart should take less than a second. This exercise will only take you one to two minutes a day if you do a complete set of 100 reps. (It sounds far more than it really is.)

> **Note:** Remember to keep your arms straight throughout the motion of pulling the band apart and stretching it.

You can also do this by raising your arms straight above your head. Keep them straight, pull the band apart with your thumbs for 100 reps. With your arms in this position, it targets your shoulders in a slightly different way.

I personally do 100 reps with my arms straight out in front of me and another 100 reps with my arms straight above.

Within a few weeks of doing these daily, you should start to see more toned shoulders, which will help make your waist look smaller.

The 5-Second Flat Belly Secret Exercise

This third and final hourglass routine is a simple five- to fifteen-second exercise that helps you reduce the size of your waist by two to three inches in less than a month. It's a foundational exercise, but for some reason few know about it. The exercise is called the Vacuum Pose.

Perhaps the simplicity of it makes some – incorrectly – assume it's no good. The fact is, it works and is the perfect example of an Effortless Exercise.

You will perform the Vacuum Pose daily for at least five minutes. Its beauty is its simplicity.

I need to warn you of something first. You *may* feel uncomfortable doing this exercise at first. But I want to encourage you to keep at it.

It's true that it is simple and the results will come fairly quickly. You can perform the vacuum pose either standing up, on your knees, sitting down, or on your hands and knees. Do what is best for *you*. Everybody is different and the position you choose has little to do with the results.

Note: I personally do the Vacuum Pose standing up (with my back against a wall) and sometimes I do it sitting down.

The Exercise

Here is how you perform the Vacuum Pose: While taking a deep breath and inhaling from your stomach (and not your chest), focus on your stomach getting sucked into your spine. In other words, literally visualize trying to pull your belly button into your spinal cord.

Now you need to maintain this pose. Keep the isometric tension in your belly region for five to 15 seconds. It's important for you to remember that this *isn't* just sucking in your stomach! It is more than that. You must see that the Vacuum Pose takes that farther.

Always focus on your lower abs and belly button when doing the Vacuum Pose. Always focus on that central part of your belly getting sucked into your spine and lower back and maintain the abdominal tension as you do the exercise.

So to recap this ultra-simple routine:

1. Suck in your lower belly in as much as possible.

2. Hold that sucked-in pose for 5-15 seconds.

3. Relax for 5-15 seconds

4. Repeat until you've done it for five full minutes.

As an alternative, you don't have to do the full five minutes all at once. Isn't that beautiful?

If you're too busy for even five minutes you can space it out over your day! Feel free to perform the Vacuum Pose here and there throughout the day. If you're really busy, just wait until you watch a TV show in the evening and do your Vacuum Pose during TV commercials.

The only reason in doing them all at once, without the television, is that to get the best results, you need to really focus while doing these. You *must* focus on your belly button getting sucked into your lower back. It seems like such a minor thing but that visualization ensures that you perform this routine exactly the way it's supposed to be done for maximum effect. That's critically important to successfully lose two to three inches from your waist in about a month.

Don't be surprised if your pants and clothes feel looser in a few weeks.

Note: Before you ever begin doing the Vacuum Pose, measure your waist (at your belly button circumference) first thing in the morning so you will know how many inches you lose the first month. Measure your waist no more than once a week to check on your progress. Your waist size is much more telling than your weight on an exercise such as the Vacuum Pose.

One final thing to remember: Be sure to do the Vacuum Pose only when you have an empty stomach.

By the Way

One last thing before we move away from the Vacuum Pose...

As I said above, your measurements are more critical than your weight. The Vacuum Pose is the best exercise you can do to take inches off your waist, but it doesn't do anything for pure weight loss on the scales. But don't worry about that.

Your goal is to look as good as possible. Your weight is secondary to that. Your weight includes water gain or loss, muscle gain or loss, and more. Your weight is not the same thing as your fat. The success of how well you conquer fat will be shown in your waist measurement and not on the scales.

As far as breathing while doing the Vacuum Pose, you can either hold your breath for the full 5-15 seconds or let out little breaths. But, if you let out little breaths you need to be sure to maintain the tension in your abdominal wall while holding the Vacuum Pose.

10
HOW TO DO HITT "RUNNING" FOR SUCCESSFUL WEIGHT LOSS

HIIT stands for *High Intensity Interval Training*. If the thought of running for hours on end sounds like a nightmare to you, you're going to like HITT Running a lot.

HITT Running is similar to the previous section's Stair Runs-Walks. The exception is that you'll be running outside (or if absolutely necessary, on a treadmill) instead of using stairs. But like the Stair Runs-Walks, you will also alternate running with walking when you perform HITT Running.

The Problems with Distance Running

"Why not simply jog at a steady pace instead of alternating between running and walking?" That is a common question. We've been told for decades that a half-hour to an hour of regular aerobic exercises is good for us. We've been told that we lose more fat if we can build up our aerobic endurance.

We've been told wrongly.

What traditional jogging, running, and other extended aerobic forms of exercises actually do is burn muscle as their source of fuel and energy.

This is *bad*! This is the last thing you want to do.

Have you ever wondered why joggers usually don't have nice bodies even after years of jogging? Think of something else. How many marathon runners actually *look* healthy?

People who exercise a lot using extended aerobic forms, such as running and jogging for distances, begin to take on a pallor that give the impression of an unhealthy appearance. This is because their bodies may very well *be* unhealthy due to all this exercise. Their bodies eat away at their muscles, which ends up giving them a pallor that might even become a soft and pudgy look.

Burning muscle is bad because the more muscle you have, the higher your *basal metabolic rate* (also known as *BMR*) is. Muscles improve your metabolism because muscles require more energy than fat. The more muscles you have the more calories burn off throughout your day. And more muscle, even if you don't exercise, means you burn more body fat than if you led the very same lifestyle without the muscle.

You *must* avoid long distance jogging because it burns off mostly muscle, not fat.

Back to HIIT Running

HIIT Running is intense and quick to do. The shortness of HITT Running helps ensure that your body has no chance to burn muscle for energy.

What HIIT Running does (in a way, the Stair Runs-Walks is a form of HIIT running) is that it produces EPOC – excess post-exercise oxygen consumption. A lot of times, EPOC is called *afterburn*.[20] Afterburn is the effect where your body continues to burn fat after you stop exercising.

By doing HIIT Running, EPOC causes an elevated rate

of calorie burning that usually lasts for hours and hours after you finished exercising. In some cases, your body still has an elevated rate of calorie burning for 18-36 hours after you finished the exercise. Talk about maximizing your exercise's effectiveness! Fat loss during the exercise is actually miniscule compared to how much fat is burns off AFTER the exercise due to it elevating your metabolism.

That's why this is so effective for fat loss. More calories get burned for more hours... even after you stop exercising. And the shock is how little effort is required to *get* to the point of EPOC.

You don't burn fat during HIIT Running exercise (don't worry about and don't even think about burning fat during exercise – it's unimportant), but immediately after doing HIIT Running, EPOC goes to work breaking down fat and releasing free fatty acids (FFA) into your blood. This results in extended fat loss.

The HITT "Running" Plan

The most effective plan for HIIT running is simply to run at between 80-90% of your top speed for five to ten seconds. After your run, you then walk for however long it takes until you feel you're fully recovered enough to run at 80-90% for another 5-10 seconds.

Keep repeating that cycle for 15 minutes and then stop.

Note: In other words, 15 minutes of running and walking can give you hours and hours of fat-burning effectiveness. That is tremendous news for those of us who have no time to spend an hour a day in the gym.

Each person is different.

Your ultimate goal should be something like running for 10 seconds and walking 50 seconds. With that routine, you'll be able to do 15 sprints of 10 seconds. This totals only two and a half minutes of total running.

That's literally all the running you'll need to do.

You will find it greatly helps to warm up with a moderate-paced walk for 5 minutes before doing HITT Running. For the fastest possible weight loss, do the HITT Running exercise four to five days a week.

Don't worry if you cannot perform the full HITT Running routine when you first begin. If you're out of shape, progress up to being able to do 10 seconds of running followed by 50 seconds of walking. You can run for five seconds and walk for 85 seconds. Keep repeating that so you'll be able to do 10 runs of 5 seconds in the 15 minutes. That's 50 seconds of running.

Once you've begun that, then it's just a matter of increasing your running times and decreasing your walking times progressively over a couple weeks. You'll work up to the full HIIT Running routine before you know it.

Note: Incidentally, for those of you who *may* want to quickly get in shape to run a 5 or 10k race, the best way is to do a modified HIIT Running program where you do a fast jog or run for as long as you can and then walk until you feel fully enough recovered to speed back up. This challenges your body without attacking your muscle stores as quickly as traditional long-distance exercising. Simply keep repeating that over a few miles several days a week. By doing that, your runs will get longer and your walks will get shorter. You'll get in better shape and better running shape a lot faster by doing that than simply jogging the whole time.

I do want to note however, that if you want to lose fat as fast as possible, don't do this modified HIIT Running. Do the Stair Runs-Walks or HIIT Running at the 15 minutes of running/walking pace.

Additional Calorie-Burning Tip

I want to add a *big tip* here on how you can burn even additional more calories.

While doing the Stair Runs-Walks or the HIIT Running routine, whether on a treadmill or outside, during the walks consciously and deliberately take big deep breaths at a pace of about one every five to ten seconds.

The reason for this is that, as you may now guess, the deep breathing floods more oxygen into your lungs and blood which causes more free fatty acids to break down and get shuttled into your blood and released out of your body. You are, in effect, amplifying the exercise's already powerful oxygen infusion by consciously controlling your breathing in this way.

11
DOING OTHER EXERCISES NOT MENTIONED HERE

If I didn't list an exercise that you like to do, there is just one thing you need to understand.

Use the "Effortless Exercise Principles" explained in this book while doing your other favorite exercises. It doesn't matter if you're doing a weight-resistance exercise, a bodyweight exercise, or cardio exercises.

You can effectively use the Effortless Exercise principles to get more and better results from that exercise. *You will maximize and leverage the work you do!*

The only limitation is your own creativity on how you use the principles.

Note that with a lot of the exercises I didn't give examples of using the Effortless Exercise System principles because I didn't want to appear redundant.

In a nutshell, with these principles you take an exercise, figure out how much of it you can do in a set (time or reps), and then cut that set in half and shorten your typical rest times between sets by more than half.

If you were to do 5 sets of 10 curls for your arms with a rest time of 1 minute between sets. Flip that using these principles so you'd do 10 sets of 5 reps resting 30 seconds (or less) between sets. This allows you to stay fresher and do more quality reps and more quality sets while improving your neural efficiency, which will allow you to add more volume quicker over the course of weeks and months... and/or cut the rest times to increase your exercise density (more exercise in less time).

This will allow you to progress faster because you eventually are able to do a lot more "easy" training that potentiates your CNS (without burdening it), which stimulates toning and weight loss.

12
THE RUNNING SUCKS EFFORTLESS EXERCISE SYSTEM SUMMARY

Working out doesn't have to be hard or take you forever. You can do short workouts or mini-workouts. Such exercises are easier to do.

They are easier to fit into your busy schedule. You will recover from them quicker. And this will allow you to do more working out overall. With the added time you put into working out, you will imprint your Nervous System and neural impulses with exercise efficiency that will get faster results for you.

The end result is you will lose weight quicker and your body will tone up a lot faster.

The great thing about all this is that you won't feel out of breath while exercising, for the most part. You'll rarely, if ever, sweat when using the Effortless Exercise principles. You won't feel like you're suffering to get a better body. With all of that, you will be more likely to work out and keep exercising.

You'll develop good exercise habits that will last years and help you to maintain a beautiful, sexy, feminine body. You *can* get a better body while exercising in a manner that seems easy. That's the Effortless Exercise way.

There is no one-way to use this information. Use it the way that is best for *you*. I'm different from you. Your friends are different from you. We all have different schedules and responsibilities and we all differ in our current abilities and stamina.

Also, we've shown you how to "break" the Effortless Exercise Method rules in an intelligent way. When you break the rules, just keep the principles in mind to maximize your results. There are many ways to burn off fat. Use the exercises and methods that work best for you. Practice and experiment.

13
OTHER STOMACH-ENHANCERS

You can build a better belly!

What an incredible belly-loving exercise we find in The Isometric Belly Squeeze!

You can perform The Isometric Belly Squeeze exercise at the same time session you're doing The Vacuum Pose. It's important to remember however that The Isometric Belly Squeeze exercise is more for toning your abs *after* your abs look pretty good already. This is why The Vacuum Pose is the best place to begin and then you add The Isometric Belly Squeeze about a month later.

With The Isometric Belly Squeeze, you are, in effect, taking your abs from looking pretty good to looking *great* with this exercise. Basically, if you're busy, you can hold off on doing this exercise until after your belly area is leaner from doing The Vacuum Pose.

The Exercise

For The Isometric Belly Squeeze, here is what you do:

1. Tighten and flex your abdominal muscles as hard as possible. Do this for 5-10 seconds.

2. Stop (release the tightness).

3. Relax for five seconds.

4. Repeat until you've performed The Isometric Belly Squeeze for five minutes.

As with The Vacuum Pose, you don't have to do The Isometric Belly Squeeze for 5 minutes straight through. You can do five seconds here and five seconds there during the day.

In fact, spacing out your sessions with The Isometric Belly Squeeze throughout the day is preferred. Your body starts to adapt to these frequent belly squeezes by staying tighter throughout the day. Soon, you will find that your abs will be tight the entire day without you even purposely trying to tighten them. It just happens naturally.

Note: Tighter abs begins to improve several other factors that you may not realize are related. Your back should tire less easily than before. Your posture probably will improve. Getting up and sitting down will be surprisingly simpler.

Make sure to perform The Isometric Belly Squeeze exercises on an empty stomach. Doing it before a meal is fine, but not afterwards.

The Isometric Belly Squeeze exercise brings a lot of definition to your entire waist and belly area. The Isometric Belly Squeeze is also great for squeezing out some of the excess water weight you're holding in your belly area.

For women, this exercise brings out the sexy, feminine toned look. For guys, it helps brings out the shredded and ripped look.

Nothing could be nicer!

How to Rub Your Belly to Burn Off Fat

Yes, by rubbing your belly you burn off fat, but only if you learn how to do the amazing routine called The Belly Rub properly.

The Belly Rub is one of the easiest ways to lose fat over the long run. The Belly Rub is *not* a quick weight-loss technique and it was never designed to be that.

It's quick just like the other two are. And The Belly Rub will only take three minutes of your time each day. And you don't even need three minutes in succession! Perform The Belly Rub for one minute each time after you eat a meal.

Note: You can literally burn fat cells out of your body using The Belly Rub.

Not only that, The Belly Rub drastically improves your digestion. Improving your digestion increases the speed of any weight loss you were doing before by making your loss more efficient.

The Belly Rub Exercise

Here's how you do The Belly Rub:

1. Take both of your hands and rub them together really fast for about five to ten seconds. This creates heat. Heat is energy. Energy burns calories.

2. While lying down (or standing up), take one of your hands and rub it in a circle around your belly button. Your hand has to touch your skin. You can't do this over your shirt.

Note: With your other hand, you can put it on your heart. Surprisingly, by putting your free hand on your heart you work to strengthen your heart with the heat energy from your hand! There is no need to move your hand in a circle over your heart.

You will rub your hand around your belly button in a circle for about 30 seconds. Use a pace of one to two circles per second.

It doesn't matter which hand or which direction

you rub.

3. After 30 seconds, stop and rub your hands together again for 5 seconds to create more heat.

4. Now, do The Belly Rub again.

Background and Insight

As I said above, rubbing your hands together creates heat and this heat is a sort of invisible kinetic energy. Basically, the heat helps to burn out fat cells from your belly area. By rubbing your hands in a circle over your belly, you also improve the digestion of food.

This teaches the body to use the food more efficiently and pull out more nutrients while properly eliminating excess food and wastes that your body doesn't need.

Note: And here's an added bonus your whole family will appreciate: The Belly Rub also helps reduce gas!

The Belly Rub causes the heat in your hands to penetrate through the skin and loosens up, breaks down, and incinerates fat deposits. Fat deposits are resilient though. So you have to repeatedly do this.

If you do this enough (and if you're consistent), eventually the fat deposits will breakdown over time and be eliminated. This technique actually goes back to ancient China, 6,000 years ago. The real shame is that simple techniques such as The Belly Rub are lost on the modern world of pills and surgery.

Follow-Up to the Belly Rub

You may still be skeptical of The Belly Rub working, but all I ask is an hour and a half of your time, spread out over a month. In other words, all I ask is for you to do The Belly Rub for one minute after each meal and do this for 30 days.

That's not asking much. You really have nothing to lose and a lot to gain.

One other thing before I wrap this up. Here are a few added thoughts (if you're a woman): If you're a woman who has heavy, painful menstrual periods, the belly rubs can help you. On the days of your period, try doing the belly rubs for up to ten minutes at a time to help relieve the pain.

The belly rubs are also beneficial for women experiencing menopause and women trying to conceive because of the improvement in circulation, lymphatic, and nerve impulses to the pelvic areas.

Bonus Belly Exercise: You Don't Have to be Hawaiian to Do This Exercise!

Hula Hooping is an additional exercise you may want to consider. Be warned, this isn't your childhood form of Hula Hooping though!

If you're looking to tone the waist and hips while helping to lose your love handles and create sexy, feminine hourglass curves, this is a great exercise. You get a lot of motion and a good return in sculpting your waistline.

How to Do This Exercise the Right Way

You want to perform every exercise properly so that you don't waste time and effort. For performing Hula Hooping properly so it's as effective as it can be, you need to get a *weighted* hula-hoop. This is *not* the kid's toy version. Be sure to get a hula-hoop that weighs two to three pounds.

Anything lighter than that and it's too hard to keep the hoop from falling to the ground. Anything heavier and it just makes hooping uncomfortable. Two to three pounds is the perfect middle ground for people to maximize their toning and shaping to bring out the hourglass curves.

If you're in the USA or Canada, you can find several options on Amazon by searching for *weighted hula hoop*. They generally cost about $30 to $40.

More Details

Now, I just want to stress this again because I don't want you to get frustrated. The *only* exercise you must do in this book to lose two to three inches from your waist in less than a month is the Vacuum Pose (if losing inches off your waist is the main goal).

As far as the Hula Hooping, you just need to do it for five to ten minutes total each day. Just like the other exercises mentioned, you don't need to do the five to ten minutes in a row, non-stop. And you don't ever need to perform all five to ten minutes during the same workout.

I personally like to do one to two minutes of Hula Hoping at a time during TV commercials (big surprise!). I do this five to six times total and then stop for the day. You can do it however you want, but if you're going to Hula Hoop, do it at least five to ten minutes a day.

The results are gradual (not fast), but you'll begin noticing a tightening and toning of your whole waist and hips area over time.

The T-Bar Kettlebell Swing

If I were to pick one single exercise to drop fat fast, for people who aren't used to exercising, without needing to leave your home, this may be it (Okay, *maybe* burpees is the fastest, but this is a close second). This is the *only* exercise you'd need to do to drop a lot of weight *and* develop a buns of steel. Yes, it's one of the fastest ways to get a killer butt.

Do I have your attention?

Below I'm showing you a picture of a kettlebell swing.

However, instead of a kettlebell, I want you to make a T-Bar Kettlebell because this allows you to adjust the weight. You won't have to buy multiple, expensive kettlebells.

A *T-Bar Kettlebell* costs about $15 to 20 in parts that you can get at Home Depot or Lowe's in the USA. If you're not in the USA, your local hardware store will have the parts you need. I'll explain more in a minute.

Here's the picture of kettlebell swings:

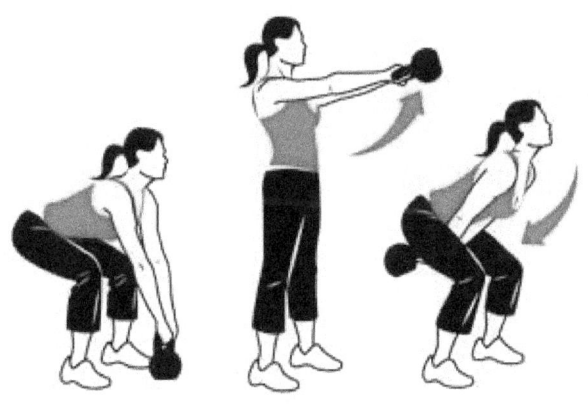

The finer points are hard to explain, but simple to show you. Instead of writing about them, I'll link you to online videos.

Tim Ferris, author of *The 4-Hour Body* has two videos. The first video shows you how to do the swings properly. The second video talks about the T-Bar Kettlebell as a cheap replacement for swings instead of kettlebells.

http://www.fourhourworkweek.com/blog/2011/01/08/kettlebell-swing/

The two keys for swings are to stick out your butt and then thrust your hips forward. You don't want to use your arms and shoulders to muscle up the weight. Use your butt and hips to power the weight up through the swinging motion.

In the picture above, the form is slightly off because she's raising the weight *slightly* too high and extending out her arms too much which will cause your arms and shoulders to muscle the weight up.

Keep watching the videos until you understand these key points so you'll know how to do swings correctly. Now, the second video doesn't give enough details on how to buy or create your own T-Bar. So I'm going to expand on that.

When you go to Home Deport or wherever to buy the parts, write this down on your list:

- A 3/4-inch x 10-12 inches long galvanized steel pipe nipple (if you are normal height or taller, go with 12 inch long pipe; if you're shorter, go with 10 inch long pipe). This will cost about $4.

- 3/4-inch by 4-5 inch long galvanized steel pipe nipple (you need to buy two, these are the handles you'll hold on to, so make sure you get two and not one). You can get a 4-inch pipe, a 4.5-inch pipe, or a 5-inch pipe. I recommend a 4.5-inch pipe if possible. That works for people with average or slightly big hands. Two of these pipes will cost $3-4 total.

- A 3/4-inch galvanized steel T coupling (this is to connect all 3 of the pipes above to each other). This costs about $2.50.

- A 3/4-inch galvanized steel Floor Flange. This will be the bottom part of the T-Bar, which will hold the weights on so they don't fly off while you're doing the swings. This will cost about $6.

- A 1-2 inch spring clamp. This will cost $2-3.

The total cost for everything is less than $20.

To put this together, all you or, a friend, need to do once you have all those parts is to screw the three pipes into the T coupling until they're tight. You only need your hands. Then screw the Floor Flange to the bottom of the 10 to 12 inch steel pipe. Make sure the Floor Flange is extremely tight. You don't want the weights flying off.

All of this takes about two minutes to do.

You can then remove the handle part by unscrewing it with your hands. Then you can slide weight plates on. That's the genius behind the T-Bar as a replacement for kettlebells. Your one T-Bar can be any weight you want it to be. You can add or remove weights as you wish.

You'll need to buy *standard* weight plates separately. I don't know how strong you are, but if you're average strength or pretty strong, you might want to start out with 10 to 15 pounds of weights. Get two 10 and 5 pound plates, each.

You can also get 25-pound standard (not Olympic-sized) weight plates from Walmart for about $20 each. I prefer you get 10 pound weights because they're smaller and easier to swing between your legs. Practice your form on the swings with just 10 to 15 pounds to begin with (or less if you feel that is too much weight).

Once you have your T-Bar Kettlebell and you have your weights, what then? Here's what I suggest you do in order to lose a lot of weight and flatten your belly:

Pick a weight, anywhere between 15 and 30 pounds and simply do 200 T-Bar swings a day for six days a week.

That's it!

Now, you can do this however you want. It doesn't matter how many swings you do per set. Just do a total of 200 swings however possible. The first few times you do this you'll probably be extremely sore. After the first day of doing 200 swings, you'll probably want to rest a day or two.

Then in two to three days, do another 200 swings. If you're really sore again, then take another one or two days off. After that, you should be able to do them every day, six days a week.

Here's how I recommend you do the 200 swings for a workout. Do them all in 15 to 20 minutes. Try to do sets of 15 swings (even if you can do a lot more). Make an effort to build up to that if you need to.

Keep doing this workout every day and trying to beat your best time. Try to get it so you do 200 swings in about 12 minutes. Once you can do that with whatever weight you were using for 200 swings in 12 minutes or less, increase the weight by 5-10 pounds.

This will make the exercise harder and it'll take you a little longer to do. But again, keep trying to beat your best time and once you can do this new weight for 200 swings in 10 to 12 minutes, increase the weight again.

Continue that progression. Also, if you're main goal is simply to lose belly fat and you're not an athlete training, I recommend that you don't go over 50 pounds with the T-Bar swings. You can if you want, but I recommend that you don't.

A second way you can do your T-Bar swings workout

is to do the swings during TV commercial breaks (I bet you heard that before!). Watch a typical one-hour or 30-minute TV show. Then during the commercials, do your swings. The typical one-hour TV show has 7 to 8 commercial breaks that last about three minutes long. So that's plenty of time to fit in 200 swings while allowing you to watch TV and without messing up you schedule.

Note: Make sure dogs, cats, wives, and children are out of the way!

The bottom line is that if you're able to do 200 T-Bar swings in 10 to 15 minutes a day, six days a week, using a decent amount of weight (25 or even more pounds), you honestly don't even need the rest of the exercises in this book in order to lose weight and belly fat.

The swings alone are all that you need. In fact, it may be best that you start out by focusing only on doing the swings and nothing else. This makes things as simple and uncluttered as possible.

You don't have to mentally think about anything else.

14
THE 1-MINUTE T-TAP

No matter how much diet and exercise training we get, there always seem to be additional little tidbits we can use to maximize our results. I wanted to give you one extra tip and something to think about.

Tap into This Gland for Additional Fat Loss

This routine is known as the *Thyroid Tap*.

The actual physical tapping of your thyroid gland (it's on the lower front part of your neck, where the "hole" in your neck is) stimulates an under-active thyroid to move towards more normalized activity.[21]

You will need to do these thyroid taps daily and for a few weeks, but it's so easy and quick that is shouldn't be a big deal to do them.

Take one or two of your fingers and tap your thyroid with your fingertips for a minute at a time a few times each day when it's convenient.

I recommend you do this tapping for a grand total of three minutes a day.

You can do it whenever and wherever, even when you're watching television, so make an effort to do them so your thyroid can get back to a normal functioning level.

An under-active thyroid (hypothyroidism) is one of the key factors that prevents people (especially women since hypothyroidism is more prevalent in women) from losing weight. Most of the time, people don't even realize they have hypothyroidism.

By tapping your thyroid for a minute at a time, you help to stimulate the thyroid into making thyroid hormones. Thus, you help your chances of losing weight because you will have a healthy, normal functioning thyroid.

If your diet is pretty good and you exercise a lot, but you're still not losing weight, your thyroid may be the thing that is holding back your progress. Give it a boost with the Thyroid Tap.

15
CONCLUDING THOUGHTS FOR
RUNNING SUCKS

As you know now, *Running Sucks* is geared toward those who either dislike the traditional endless running and aerobics, or for those who simply don't have time to devote to those hours and hours of activity. Plus, it turns out that endless hours of daily aerobics types of exercises are not the most efficient or the most effective ways to approach fat loss and toning.

Interval kinds of training such as HITT, as well as approaches such as Tabata are far superior. Plus, they take far less time and in this modern, busy time isn't that what we all need? As long as you follow the approaches in this book, you should steadily lose the fat and tone your thighs and hips and belly.

The concepts in *Running* Sucks work exceptionally well when you combine them with our *10-Hour Coffee Diet*. that you can get here: http://www.amazon.com/10-Hour-Coffee-Diet-Transform-Health-ebook/dp/B00HB77U44/

We wish you *only good fortune* in your body sculpting. More important, we wish you the best health possible. Good luck and we hope to hear about your weight loss and health transformation.

Sincerely,

Jennifer Jolan and Rich Bryda

REFERENCES

1 *"Whirling Dervishes,"*
http://en.wikipedia.org/wiki/Mevlevi_Order

2 *"Five Tibetan Rites,"*
http://www.mkprojects.com/pf_TibetanRites.htm

3 *"The Endocrine System,"*
http://en.wikipedia.org/wiki/Endocrine_system

4 *"Human Homeostasis,"*
http://en.wikipedia.org/wiki/Human_homeostasis

5 *"THE EVOLUTION, STRUCTURE AND FUNCTION OF THE NERVOUS SYSTEM - Imprinting is a Single-flash Exposure of the Neural Film which Defines and Limits the Neuro-umbilical Reality,"*
http://www.oocities.org/elishamcmears/ip-1-16.html

6 *"How to Get Stronger at Push-ups and Pull-ups Using a Soviet Special Forces Technique,"*
http://fitnessblackbook.com/strength-training/how-to-get-stronger-at-push-ups-and-pull-ups-using-a-soviet-special-forces-technique/

7 *"Hebbian Theory,"*
http://en.wikipedia.org/wiki/Hebbian_theory

8 *"Brain activity of Normal and Low IQ children: The neural efficiency hypothesis,"*
http://www.academia.edu/5304180/Brain_activity_of_

Normal and Low IQ children The neural efficiency hypothesis

[9] *"Central Nervous System,"* http://www.nlm.nih.gov/medlineplus/ency/article/002311.htm

[10] *"Speeding up central nervous system recovery,"* http://forum.bodybuilding.com/showthread.php?t=119731301

[11] *"Human Growth Hormone (HGH),"* http://www.webmd.com/fitness-exercise/human-growth-hormone-hgh

[12] *"Training To Failure: A Look Inside,"* http://www.weighttrainer.net/training/failure.html

[13] *"The Bulgarian Method of Training Olympic Weightlifters,"* http://startingstrength.com/resources/forum/showthread.php?t=23348

[14] *"High Intensity Interval Training – The Tabata Protocol,"* http://www.brianmac.co.uk/tabata.htm

[15] *"8 Benefits of High-Intensity Interval Training (HIIT),"* http://www.shape.com/fitness/workouts/8-benefits-high-intensity-interval-training-hiit

[16] *"The Best Exercise For Your Immune System: Rebounding!,"* http://www.chrisbeatcancer.com/rebounding/

[17] *"Extreme Endurance Exercise: If You Do This Type of Exercise, You Could Be Damaging Your Heart,"* http://fitness.mercola.com/sites/fitness/archive/2013/08/23/extreme-endurance-exercise.aspx

[18] *"Adenosine Triphosphate,"* http://hyperphysics.phy-astr.gsu.edu/hbase/biology/atp.html

[19] *"What Is Cellulite? What Causes Cellulite?,"* http://www.medicalnewstoday.com/articles/149465.php

[20] *"Afterburn Effect: Burn 500+ Calories from 10 Minutes of Exercise?,"* http://www.builtlean.com/2011/06/29/afterburn-effect-of-exercise-qa-with-dr-christopher-scott-phd/

[21] *"The Thyroid Gland,"* http://umm.edu/programs/diabetes/health/endocrinology-health-guide/thyroid-gland